CIVILIZATION AND DISEASE

Civilization
and Disease

Henry E. Sigerist

Phoenix Books

THE UNIVERSITY OF CHICAGO PRESS

CHICAGO & LONDON

PHOENIX SCIENCE SERIES

THE UNIVERSITY OF CHICAGO PRESS, CHICAGO & LONDON
The University of Toronto Press, Toronto 5, Canada

Preface

THE PRESENT BOOK is based on a series of six Messenger Lectures that I delivered at Cornell University in Ithaca in November and December 1940. I am very much indebted to the authorities of the University and Press for the permission to develop the six lectures into a book of twelve chapters, and I also very much appreciate the patience they have shown in waiting for a much delayed manuscript.

While I was writing this book, I relived the very pleasant weeks it was my privilege to spend on the Cornell campus, and I am deeply grateful to the authorities of the University, to faculty and students for the delightful hospitality extended to me. I wish to mention particularly the keen and enthusiastic members of the Telluride Association whose guest I was during my visit. I shall always remember with great pleasure the stimulating discussions we had on many an evening.

The subject of this book is one in which I have been interested for many years. In the pursuit of these studies I was greatly encouraged by Dr. Ludwig Kast, the unforgettable first President of the Josiah Macy Jr. Foundation, with whom I discussed these problems many times and through whom I obtained a substantial grant from the Josiah Macy Jr. Foundation which made it possible to acquire source materials needed for this book, and for which I wish to express my profound gratitude.

And finally I wish to thank my co-workers, the members of my staff and particularly Dr. Erwin H. Ackerknecht, for advice and criticism; Genevieve Miller, my former student and present collaborator who took a very active part in the preparation of this

v

PREFACE

book; Hope Trebing and Janet Brock who helped to get the manuscript ready for publication. I am much indebted to Mr. Harold
Ward in New York, who read the manuscript critically and greatly
improved it with valuable suggestions.

Henry E. Sigerist

The Johns Hopkins Institute
of the History of Medicine
August, 1942

Contents

CONTENTS

Illustrations

Introduction

THE MESSENGER LECTURES deal with the *Evolution of Civilization,* and there can be no doubt that in this evolution disease has played a considerable part. No two phenomena could possibly be more different than disease, a material process, and civilization, the most sublime creation of the human mind. And yet the relationship between the two is very obvious.

Disease, as we conceive it today, is a biological process. The human organism responds to normal stimuli with normal physiological reactions. It possesses a high degree of adaptability to changing conditions. We can live in good health at sea level and on high altitudes, in the heat of the tropics and in the cold of the arctic, at rest and in performance of violent exercise. Our organism is able to adjust its respiration, circulation, metabolism and other functions to changing conditions—up to a certain limit. When stimuli exceed in quantity or quality the adaptability of the organism, its reactions are no longer normal but abnormal or pathological. They are symptoms of disease, functions of injured organs, or defense mechanisms that tend to overcome lesions. Disease is no more than the sum total of abnormal reactions of the organism or its parts to abnormal stimuli.

To the individual, however, disease is not only a biological process but also an experience, and it may well be one that very deeply affects his entire life. Since man is the creator of civilization, disease, by affecting his life and actions, has influence on his creations also.

Disease, moreover, sometimes attacks not merely single indi-

1

viduals but entire groups; either temporarily in epidemics, or for long periods of time in endemics, when a disease has taken firm hold on a group or region. The cultural life of such groups cannot but reflect the influence of the disease, as will be shown in many examples.

The investigation of human and animal remains of early historic and prehistoric times has demonstrated that disease was prevalent not only throughout the history of civilization but also long before the advent of man. We can safely assume that disease is as old as life itself, because there have always been stimuli that exceeded the adaptability of any organism. The examination of fossil bones has further shown that diseases have occurred at all times in the same basic forms as are encountered today. In other words, the animal organism is equipped with only a limited number of mechanisms such as inflammation, growth, etc., for effectively responding to abnormal stimuli.

Since disease has occurred at all times, all human institutions have been affected by it and have had to reckon with it in one way or another. The law, endeavoring to regulate relations between men and men and between men and things, was forced to take the sick man into account. Without approaching the problems set by disease and suffering, religion and philosophy could not explain the world, nor could literature and art have adequately recreated it. And the conquest of disease was always an important part of the attempt to master nature through science.

There is, however, another and totally different aspect of the problem. Two factors are always involved in the genesis of disease: man and his environment. Every individual is the product of the fusion of two parental cells from which he receives two sets of chromosomes, each containing genes or hereditary factors. The material with which a man must face the world is given to him once and for all at the moment of conception, and half of this material he will pass on to every one of his children. Heredity, therefore, is

2

an extremely important factor in our life. It controls to a large extent an individual's physical appearance, his longevity, intelligence, even his character and aptitudes; and it also has great influence in determining the diseases to which he will be subject during the course of his life.

Heredity, however, is not the inexorable fate that many believe it to be. Far from it. Man's equipment is given to him, but he can use it well or badly, can improve or damage it. He can, within limits, alter his physical appearance; inclined to be stout by heredity, he may through diet and exercise keep his weight down. He can develop whatever intelligence and aptitudes he has but may also waste them. He can lengthen his span of life through a rational mode of living but may also shorten it by abuse. He can overcome certain traits of his character, as, for instance, by learning to control an inherited irascibility. Thus we see that there is not only a hereditary disposition to diseases, but also an acquired one, which is determined largely by the mode of living.

At this point cultural factors enter the scene. Religion, philosophy, education, social and economic conditions—whatever determines a man's attitude towards life—will also exert great influence on his individual disposition to diseases and the importance of these cultural factors is still more evident when we consider the environmental causes of disease.

From the moment of conception, human life unfolds itself in an environment which is always both physical and social. The embryo, well protected in a narrow world under constant physical conditions, develops from the very beginning in social relationship to another individual, its mother. In this close intercourse it may be injured or infected, and when this happens the infant is born suffering from a congenital (not "hereditary") disease. As the child grows up, his environment expands. First it was the home, either in the city with its streets, or on the farm with its surrounding countryside. Then he reaches school age and he enters a new world; gradually detaching himself from the family, the original social unit, he is exposed to strong new influences. The environment broadens again when he begins to work for a living, assumes responsibilities as a citizen, and founds a new social unit.

The social and physical environment which is responsible for most diseases, is in turn shaped by the civilization that has so profoundly altered man's life. We no longer follow the rhythm of nature, awaking at sunrise and going to sleep at sunset. We have created the means of lighting up the darkness and can heat our dwellings to the temperature of summer in the middle of winter. We have learned to produce our food in the quantity and quality desired, sometimes even in complete disregard of the seasons. We have tremendously increased the speed of our communications and have extended our memory by the arts of writing and printing. We have become conscious not only of ourselves but also of our history. We are for the most part monogamous and remain deeply attached to our families throughout life. And we are trying —not always successfully—to live in peace in large social groups.

Civilization, in the course of its evolution, has often produced conditions detrimental to health. With its advantages have come many hazards and the responsibility for many diseases. The fire that warms us and cooks our food also burns and destroys; every new tool was dangerous until we had learned to handle it safely. And every tool can be used for good or evil.

Civilization created also medicine and public health. It has forged the weapons to fight disease. When man learned to direct and aid the natural fertility of the soil, agriculture was born. And when he learned to direct and aid the natural healing power of the organism, medicine was born. From being empirical, agriculture became scientific, and the healing art became medical science. Civilization eliminated many health hazards, was able to reduce considerably the incidence of many diseases and to lengthen the average span of human life.

4

These few introductory remarks suffice to show that the relationship between civilization and disease is extremely complex. The following chapters will discuss, although in no sense exhaustively, some of the major aspects of this relationship and the many problems arising from it.

CHAPTER I

Civilization as a Factor in the Genesis of Disease

CIVILIZATION is very young. For a half million years man lived like a beast in the woods, his body covered with hair, grubbing for food and sleeping in caves. At this stage he undoubtedly was subject to accidents and also to certain diseases, just as wild animals are today.

Civilization began when man discovered the use of fire, learned how to cut stone implements and to use the fur of animals as a protection against the cold. In the cave which now was lighted up by fire he sometimes painted pictures in ochre of the animals that were the objects of his hunting: the reindeer, the bison and even the mammoth. Was it to placate the spirits of the animals killed, or to fascinate them, or was it just done playfully? Who can tell?

The greatest step in the history of civilization was taken during the transition from the paleolithic to the neolithic period, when man learned to grow the plants he wanted for food, and to domesticate animals that would work for him and provide him with meat. He made baskets from willow rods and when the idea occurred to him to toughen these baskets with a layer of clay, pottery was invented. Tools became articulated and these improved tools made him independent of the cave. Now he could fell trees and build shelters. A tree hollowed out was a boat, and a boat on wheels was a cart. At this time also he probably learned to articulate his words by adding to them prefixes and suffixes, thus acquiring better means of expressing himself. Families joined to form larger social groups, living and working together, following definite sets of rules. These groups exchanged their goods for those of others and thus trade developed.

All these tremendous developments must have affected the incidence of illness among our progenitors. Many hazards were reduced; the supply of food was more secure, and the protection against cold and enemies was better. On the other hand it is very possible that the natural resistance of man was reduced largely because of an increasing dependence on the products of civilization.

Food, clothing, housing, occupation, social relations—these factors have always played a considerable rôle, both in health and disease. Let us examine them briefly, beginning with food.

Man requires oxygen and food to maintain his life. Since the air contains oxygen in unlimited quantities, it is easily available and a lack of oxygen will occur only under unusual circumstances. Food is required by the organism in a minimum quantity and in certain forms, and to obtain it man has had to exert himself strenuously. "In the sweat of thy face shalt thou eat bread." Since self-preservation and preservation of the species are the most potent drives in life, the craving for food and the sex urge were always the most powerful stimulations.

If the minimum of food needed to replace the energy spent is unavailable, man's resistance to disease is lessened, and prolonged starvation ultimately leads to death. The history of famines is a sad chapter in the history of mankind,[1] the more so since it is not yet closed. The world can produce much more food than its two-billion inhabitants require, and with the present methods of agriculture and means of communication there is no justification and no excuse for a famine. Whenever such an event occurs, it shows that civilization has somewhere collapsed.

7

Conditions were different in past centuries when the specter of hunger was ever present. The soil produced less than today. Means of transportation were slow. Regular importation of food was possible only in colonial empires where, as in ancient Rome there was a strongly organized state power. Such imports were often made at the expense of the subjugated colonial people. For thousands of years entire populations were constantly at the mercy of the weather. Failure of the crops affected the people not only directly by creating a scarcity of food, but also indirectly through unemployment and its resulting poverty. Crop failures always raised the prices of agricultural products so that the poor, made poorer by unemployment, were hit hardest.

At all times famines have led to social disturbances. In mere self-preservation people took food wherever they could find it, or stole the money to buy it. Criminality, brigandage, and prostitution were well known symptoms of famines. Families were torn apart and children grew up without guidance, as in the Russian famine of 1921, when the hordes of vagrant children presented a serious problem. Exasperated by starvation, people were ready to rise against the authorities. The sight of rich families indulging in luxuries while they were deprived of the bare necessities made them acutely aware of class distinctions. Hunger was one factor that contributed to unleash revolutionary forces in France in 1789. The Roman emperors well knew that the best way to keep the masses quiet was to give them *panem et circenses*, food and entertainment—and usually, the more entertainment, the less food. In the 2nd century after Christ about 500,000 inhabitants of Rome lived on public charity.[2] The emperors' example has been followed by all dictators.

Famines always provided a fertile breeding ground for many diseases. The lack of food not only produced oedemas and specific deficiency diseases among the people, but also, by lessening their resistance, made them an easy prey to all kinds of infections. Since famines disorganized normal life, people's living conditions became worse. The louse thrived and typhus spread. Disorganization of water supplies and food control resulted in epidemics of typhoid, dysentery and cholera. The chronicles of the plague usually report that epidemics began with drought and famine somewhere in the East, in China or India. The process is easy to understand. A drought led to crop failure. The granaries were empty. The rats and other rodents moved closer to man, and if there happened to be plague among the rodents there were good chances that the disease would be transmitted to people. And then it spread from man to man like wild-fire.

Conditions are made worse by the fact that famines set large groups of people in motion. This was not felt so much in the past when there was less freedom of movement. The mediaeval serf had no other choice than to starve on the spot. In recent famines, however, particularly in the Russian famine mentioned before, people abandoned their homes and moved into other districts that had been less afflicted. In so doing they spread whatever epidemic diseases they had.

Hunger or the threat of it were the causes of many migrations of nations. Fertile countries like the valley of the Nile or Mesopotamia were tempting goals for less privileged nations. Once every thousand years the Semitic tribes of the Arabian peninsula invaded the territory of their neighbors. Scarcity of food united the Arabic tribes under the leadership of Mohammed and his successors and was the driving force of their conquests. Hunger drove Germanic tribes into the fertile plains of Italy in the 5th century A. D. On a smaller scale we find that failure of the potato crop in 1846–1847 drove thousands of Irishmen to the United States.

The history of Europe records many famines which sometimes were local and sometimes universal. Such universal famines occurred in 879 and 1162. A famine in England in 1586 gave rise to the Poor Law System. For centuries in Russia, famines occurred on an average of once every ten years and serious crop failures once every five years until, after the Revolution, agriculture was organized along scientific lines. In India, where five-sixths of the population depend on agriculture for a living, the slightest crop failure has tremendous repercussions.[3] The famine of 1770 in Bengal killed one-third of the population. One million people succumbed to the famine of 1899–1901, and the history of China up to 1916 is full of reports of even greater catastrophes caused by lack of food.[4]

From the time of Charlemagne to the Industrial Revolution the population of Europe increased very slowly. It was determined by the productivity of the soil. This changed with the introduction of the machine. Improved means of transportation permitted an increase of population beyond the natural capacity of the soil. From then on famines were man-made, the result of mismanagement, war and blockade. For centuries wars were contests between ruling houses and were fought by professional armies. From the Napoleonic era on they became struggles between nations, and the starving out of the enemy country became one of the most popular war measures. Paris was starving in 1871, Germany and her allies in 1917–1918, and nobody knows just how far the famine caused by the present war will spread or what proportions it will assume.

In the civilized countries of the West acute famines are now relatively rare, being largely concomitant with major historical events. There is, however, another form of starvation that is worldwide and which occurs even in some of the most highly industrialized countries. It is not spectacular, not acute, but like an endemic disease it saps the vitality of the people. This form of starvation goes under the name of *malnutrition*. Its causes are primarily social and economic and, to a minor extent, lack of education. Let me give a few examples from my own experience in various countries.

The natives of South Africa, seven-tenths of the total population, are negroes, members of the large Bantu family. They used to be farmers and warriors and owned large herds of cattle. Their diet consisted chiefly of milk, mealie meal (ground African corn), and various herbs, a combination that gave them a well balanced diet. The white man took the land and exploited the natives, using them as farm laborers who sharecropped miserably on his large estates; or he gave them small parcels of land on the native reserves—usually not more than ten acres a household when land was available. Bantu economy still is a cattle economy, a man's social standing being reckoned not by the quality but by the number of cattle which he owns. In consequence, the little land available is overstocked, and cannot feed the cattle. The cow has no milk, the ox is too weak to pull the plow, and the mealie grows in insufficient quantity. The situation became worse when the government encouraged the people to raise sheep. These animals destroyed the pastures by excessive close cropping and when the mistake was recognized it was already too late. Furthermore, sheep to the native had become ready cash; something to be traded in whenever he was in want. Another complication developed when, in contact with the white people the natives discarded the herbs that they used to eat, before they had learned to grow and to prepare vegetables.

As a result of all these developments, the natives of South Africa are extremely poor. Malnutrition with all its dire consequences is the rule, and health conditions are very bad. Over 50 per cent. of all the children born never reach the age of fifteen. In the Transkeian Territory, a native reserve with a population of 1.3 million, it has been estimated that 12 pregnancies are needed for a woman to have 2 surviving children. Eight pregnancies end in miscarriage, 4 children are born, of which at least 2 die young.

Some of the Balkan countries have probably the best agricultural land of Europe, and yet in all of them the peasant population

11

is poor, undernourished and in ill health. General death rates and infant mortality rates are extremely high, as may be seen from the following table:

1931–1935	General Death Rate per 1,000 population	Infant Mortality Rate per 1,000 children born
Roumania	20.6	182
Yugoslavia	17.9	153
Greece	16.5	122
Hungary	15.8	157
Bulgaria	15.5	147

The Yugoslavian peasant before the war produced great quantities of excellent milk, butter, cheese, eggs and probably the best poultry in Europe, but he himself lived on corn-bread and beans. In order to pay his taxes he was forced to sell his products, which were mostly exported in exchange for imports that did not benefit the mass of the people. The distribution of land was very uneven. Ninety-five per cent. of all peasant families together possess less than one-half, and five per cent. somewhat more than half of the cultivated soil.[5] Most farm families that owned land had not more than eight acres of which two are needed for the sustenance of one individual.

In Roumania, the peasants constituting the overwhelming majority of the population, were for the first time in a generation well nourished when the depression was at its peak. There was no market for farm products and the peasants ate the food they produced. As a result they could not pay taxes and the chief sufferers were the legion of employees on the government payroll.

All such conditions are the result not of natural but of man-made catastrophes. They follow from the character of a civilization that was developed for the benefit of a few at the expense of the mass of the people. It is a sad commentary on our civilization that after

5,000 years we have not yet learned to supply all human beings with the food their organism requires. We have the scientific knowledge necessary for such a purpose. We know how to increase the fertility of the soil and to improve crops in quantity and quality. But when it comes to the distribution of food we discard science and let things take their course: or we think we have done our share when we distribute a little food as a measure of relief.

Food is the basic need of man, and whoever works and thus contributes to the life of society has a right to the quantity and quality of food that his organism requires. In the past, people accepted famines and malnutrition with resignation, believing them to come from forces that were beyond human control. After two centuries of enlightenment and liberal democratic government this attitude is changing rapidly. We are beginning to realize that there is no justification for being starved or undernourished in the midst of plenty. We see that this is the inevitable consequence of a social organization that can and must be changed. Even as this book is being written the world is passing through one of its greatest crises, a crisis one of whose major issues undoubtedly is the struggle for social security, for the right to work and the right to eat.

If lack of food is an important cause of disease, too much food is also harmful to health. You sometimes hear that more people die from overeating than from starvation. This is a very superficial statement, usually made by well-to-do city people who have never been hungry nor ever seen conditions in the slums of the cities or in poor rural districts. There is no doubt that overeating is harmful to the gastro-intestinal tract, and that excessive weight burdens the circulatory organs. The number of people, however, who are exposed to the danger of repletion is negligible compared to those who suffer from malnutrition.

Food habits have greatly improved, particularly since the war of 1914–1918. Restrictions due to a war economy proved beneficial in many instances and corroborated the postulates of the science of nutrition. Gluttony is no longer fashionable, and the rich man's meals have become much simpler than they had been in previous centuries when *embonpoint* was a sign of prosperity and conferred social prestige.

As a rule, the diet of a wealthy Greek was frugal [6] and still more that of the Roman at the time of the republic. Conditions changed in imperial Rome when delicacies were imported from all over the ancient world.[7] A regular dinner had seven courses, hors d'oeuvres, three entrées, two roasts, and dessert. In the Middle Ages many monasteries and courts of noblemen were renowned for the richness of their food. For centuries intemperance in eating was not frowned upon but taken for granted as the rich man's privilege. The nobles set an example that the middle class followed only too eagerly as soon as it could afford opulent living, and to the peasants and city artisans a wedding or a wake was an opportunity to eat as much as the stomach could hold, or even more. The Dutch painters of the 17th century reveled in picturing rich food in large quantities. An English country gentleman's dinner in 1768 included: [8]

A roasted Shoulder of Mutton and a plum Pudding—Veal Cutlets, Frill'd Potatoes, cold Tongue, Ham and cold roast Beef, and eggs in their shells. Punch, Wine, Beer and Cyder for drinking.

And when the same Rev. James Woodforde gave an "elegant" dinner in 1774, it consisted of the following: [8]

The first course was, part of a large Cod, a Chine of Mutton, some Soup, a Chicken Pye, Puddings and Roots, etc. Second course, Pidgeons and Asparagus. A Fillet of Veal with Mushrooms and high Sauce with it, rosted Sweetbreads, hot Lobster, Apricot Tart and in the Middle a Pyramid of Syllabubs and Jellies. We had Dessert of Fruit after Dinner, and Madeira, White Port and red to drink as Wine.

A dinner served at the United States Hotel in Saratoga Springs in August, 1890, included: [9]

OYSTERS ON HALF SHELL

SAUTERNE

GREEN TURTLE SOUP   OLIVES

BOILED SALMON   LOBSTER SAUCE   POTATO BALLS

SAUTERNE

SWEETBREAD CUTLETS   PEAS

CLARET

FILLET OF BEEF   MUSHROOM SAUCE

LIMA BEANS   MASHED POTATOES

CHAMPAGNE

ROMAN PUNCH

SUPRÊME OF CHICKEN   TRUFFLE SAUCE

TERRAPIN   SARATOGA CHIPS

PARTRIDGES ON TOAST   SALTED ALMONDS

LETTUCE   CHEESE   CRACKERS

ROQUEFORT AND NEUFCHÂTEL

ICES   MERINGUES   FRUITS

COFFEE   CIGARS   BENEDICTINE

Today such a dinner would not be considered a treat but a torture. People have become conscious of calories, and fashion requires them to be slim. While millions of poor people starve all over the world for lack of food, many rich people starve voluntarily for the sake of fashion.

Overeating is not a menace of any social significance. The excessive use of intoxicating beverages, however, is a far more serious threat, because it affects all classes.

It is interesting to note that the preparation of fermented liquors can be traced back to remotest antiquity. This art seems to be as old as agriculture itself and must have been invented spontaneously all over the globe. Beer made from malted grain was very popular in Egypt and Babylonia, and also wine, made from grapes in Egypt,

from dates in Babylonia. Grape wine frequently flavored with various spices was the fermented drink of Greece and Rome. The Greeks mixed water with it, not only to make it lighter, but also less sweet. In northern Europe before the introduction of the vine, mead was made from wild honey, and in the Far East a fermented liquor was prepared from rice.

The desire for alcoholic liquors and their universal popularity were due to various reasons. They were, first of all, consumed as food. Bread and beer were the poor man's food in Egypt; in Babylonia beer was given in part payment of wages. These liquors were a pleasant food because they had a good taste and because their alcoholic content, although moderate, was high enough to remove inhibitions so that the effect was felt as stimulating.

The use of fermented liquors also had a place in most ancient cults, from the cult of Osiris to that of Dionysus and eventually of the Christian church. Wine affects man's mind, loosens the tongue, is apt to create "enthusiasmos." Red wine has the color of life-substance, blood, and thus became its symbol. The transformation of dead vegetable and animal parts into living substance appeared as a mystery, and the act of eating assumed ritual significance. Before meals the Greek and the Roman sacrificed to the gods, the Christian said grace. Meals taken in communion under observation of certain rites were institutions found in all ancient civilizations from the Greek *symposium* to the Christian *agape*. And in these rites wine played an important part.

Drunkenness occurred occasionally wherever alcoholic liquors were consumed. It was usually accepted and taken for granted; objections, when they were made, being more for aesthetic than for moral or hygienic reasons. Southern people are, as a rule, temperate, and habitual drunkenness is rather rare in wine countries. Alcoholism became a serious health problem after man had learned to distill the "spirit of wine." The process of distillation was known in antiquity, but it was not until the 13th century that it was ap-

16

plied more commonly and then chiefly in the preparation of drugs. The highly concentrated alcoholic drinks, the "hard liquors," became a danger because they provided an easy, quick and relatively cheap means of escaping unpleasant realities.

Drinking has, in my opinion, two main causes. One is social and economic. Misery, poor living conditions, lack of educational and recreational facilities drive a man into drinking. In Russia, in 1913, the annual consumption of vodka amounted to 8.1 liters or more than 2 gallons per person, and the average worker spent over a quarter of his wages on liquor. When conditions of the working population changed after the Revolution the per capita consumption of liquor dropped steadily. It was 4.5 liters in 1931, 3.7 in 1935.[10]

Whenever people are hard pressed by a sense of misery and oppression, the more will they be inclined to seek oblivion in drink. And the more they take to drinking, the more oppressed and wretched they become. The white man's conquests owe as much to fire-water as to firearms. The effect of alcohol on the American Indian is well known. The stimulant he used was tobacco, which is not intoxicating. Whisky broke his resistance and made him an easy prey for exploitation. The same methods of conquest were applied in other parts of the world.

Another cause of harmful drinking is to be sought in folk customs and group habits. Since alcohol removes inhibitions and makes people talk more freely, it became the custom to drink alcoholic liquors whenever people gathered for social intercourse. This *alcoholisme mondain,* as the French call it, affects the most highly educated classes. It is not so spectacular, but has nevertheless very deleterious results.

Experience has shown that alcoholism cannot be overcome by prohibitions which inadvertently glorify drinking. Improved social and economic conditions leading to a greater social security will remove a main cause of drunkenness and thus make possible a radical change in customs and habits. The process is slow but entirely feasible and, as a matter of fact, progress has already been made. Young people are more conscious of health and enjoy physical exercise much more than in the past. Man will never be perfect; he will not and should not live merely for the sake of preserving his health. There will always be a desire for stimulants to compensate for the monotony and fatigues in everyday life; this need can legitimately be satisfied with drinks such as beer and wine, which, when consumed in moderate quantities, have no harmful effects.

In other parts of the world various narcotics, such as opium, hashish, *peyote* have played a rôle similar to that of alcohol. Stimulating but non-intoxicating drugs—notably those in tea, coffee, and tobacco—have become popular throughout the world. Used immoderately they are all harmful, but some of them have had very beneficial effects. The universal custom of drinking tea in China has forced the people to boil their drinking water and has thus prevented many intestinal diseases.

Dietetics was highly developed in antiquity. Some of the best Hippocratic writings are concerned with it and discuss in great detail the qualities and effects of various foodstuffs. The modern science of nutrition, however, is very young. The pioneer in the field was the chemist, Justus von Liebig (1803–1873), whose discoveries in organic chemistry were applied in agriculture and cattle breeding long before human physiology paid any attention to them. In 1873 the great hygienist Max von Pettenkofer made the characteristic statement: [11]

> It is a remarkable fact that today almost every educated farmer knows exactly how much protein and other substances he must feed to a hog, a sheep, a cow or an ox, if he wants to produce a definite result. He knows what composition of fodder is required

18

for maintenance, for fattening, for the production of milk or for muscular development. Man, however, has hardly been touched by the rays of the rising sun of the science of nutrition.

Studies on plant and animal nutrition were readily encouraged, for their advantages were easily apparent. But there was a definite opposition to their extension to human nutrition. Such studies seemed futile, for it was believed that, unlike animals, man was intelligent and knew what was good for him. The human race had survived for hundreds of thousands of years, and had thrived without any knowledge of calories. Instinctively all people had found the food that they needed and that was most appropriate to the climate in which they lived. And to many people it also seemed degrading to draw close parallels between animals and man.

Pettenkofer had a very pertinent answer to these objections.[12] There can be no greater difference, he said, than that between the soul of a nursing mother and a cow, but the milk they both produce is very similar, so much so that one can be used for the other. We feed children with cow's milk and it would be possible to raise a calf on mother's milk. Rich people can buy all the food they want in any combination and quality they please. But the poor who can obtain only a minimum—what food should they buy preferably? Or the soldiers and inmates of prisons and asylums who have little or no choice—what food should be given to them so as to keep them in good health? There was, Pettenkofer concluded, a definite need for nutritional standards and only physiological research could establish them.

A student of Liebig and co-worker of Pettenkofer, Carl Voit, did pioneer service in the field. One of his students, Max Rubner, continued these studies very successfully. In recent years the science of nutrition has been highly developed in America. The discovery of the vitamins was particularly significant. Dreaded maladies such as rickets, scurvy, beriberi and pellagra were found to be deficiency diseases, or those caused by the *lack* of a definite vitamin. It became possible to cure and prevent them.

Here, as in so many cases, experience preceded science. Scurvy was the curse of navigation. It attacked crews and passengers of sailing vessels, producing many casualties, and sometimes even wrecking entire expeditions. Long before vitamin C was discovered, it was known that fresh fruits and vegetables cured and prevented scurvy. As early as the 17th century, Dutch boats sailing to the East Indies carried large supplies of oranges,[13] and lime juice became a staple food on British sailing vessels. In 1711 a Dutch physician, Abraham Bogaert, wrote the prophetic words: [14]

> I wished my colleagues who discourse so prolixly about the treatment of this disease would recognize that the grass in the fields, inconspicuous as it is, has a greater power to heal this disease than all their fancied wisdom and unsurpassed panaceas.

Today we know what a wholesome and well-balanced diet should be. If there is still an enormous amount of malnutrition in the world, lack of education must share the blame with the social and economic factors that are primarily responsible. Food habits are determined by old traditions, and are therefore very tenacious and hard to change. Education has a particularly difficult task in this field because faulty diet is not a conspicuous killer, nor does it lead to immediate illness. It makes people unfit and prepares the ground for the development of disease. The need for changing a traditional diet thus is not always apparent. We still have a long way to go.

In the history of *clothing* and of its effects on health we must differentiate between climates. In the tropics there is no physical need for clothes; people can live nude, and if they dress it is not for protection. In the arctic, on the other hand, the body is covered completely as a measure of protection and in order to reduce

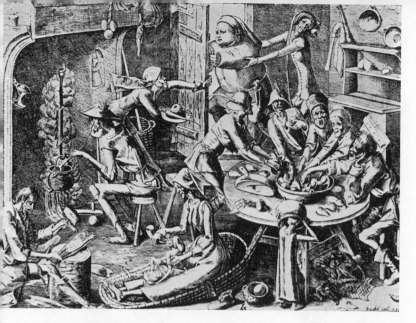

1. STARVATION. Engraving by Peter Breughel the Elder, 1563.

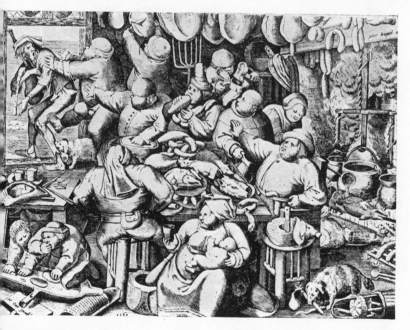

2. GLUTTONY. Engraving by Peter Breughel the Elder, 1563. (Both pictures by the courtesy of the Baltimore Museum of Art.)

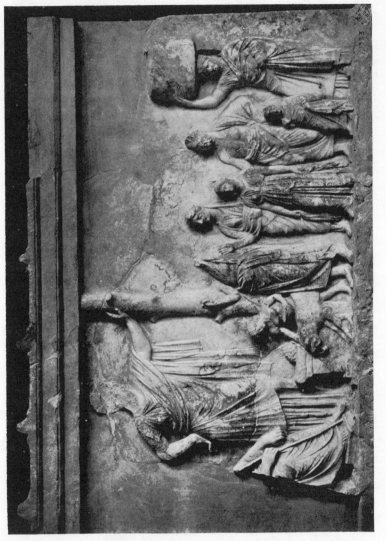

3. GREEK COSTUMES. Asclepius, Hygeia, and suppliants. (Votive relief from Asclepius temple of Athens, end of 5th or 4th century B.C.)

the loss of body heat. In the temperate zones in which we live, clothing serves a variety of purposes.

The Bible attributes the custom of dressing to the original sin: [15]

> And the eyes of them both were opened, and they knew that they were naked; and they sewed fig leaves together, and made themselves aprons.
>
> Unto Adam also and to his wife did the Lord God make coats of skins, and clothed them.

This interpretation is correct in so far as it implies that modesty was originally unknown to man; that it is secondary, a product of civilization. It is wrong in that it reverses the order by assuming that modesty suggested the fig leaf rather than followed the act of wearing it.

In the animal kingdom nature has frequently made the male much more conspicuous than the female. The lion has a mane, the cock a comb and gorgeous plumage. What nature denied to the human male he acquired for himself as civilization developed. Paint, tattoo, ornamental scars preceded regular clothing and were employed by men sooner and more often than by women. The purpose was obviously to create a sexual stimulus, and in certain cases also to denote an individual's rank, or it had magical significance.

A next step was taken when man began to adorn his body with foreign objects, with necklaces, bracelets, rings and similar ornaments—and with clothes. These subjects were worn for decoration and frequently, but not exclusively, as amulets for protection against evil spirits and the evil eye. Clothes were worn to conceal certain parts of the body and thus to draw attention to them. Their primary purpose was that of a sexual stimulant.

The original dress of tropical regions was the girdle [16] which developed into the loin cloth, the skirt and, when suspended on the shoulders, into the shirt and the cloak. When man migrated north and clothing had to serve also as a protection against the cold, trousers developed, probably from the loin cloth. The trousers became the characteristic arctic dress. Among the Eskimos both men and women wear them. In tropical Africa both sexes wear girdles or skirts. In Greece and Rome the tropical dress prevailed and consisted basically of skirt and cloak, *chiton* or *peplos* and *himation, tunica* and *pallium.* Only northern barbarians were known to wear trousers.

Changes occurred in Europe in the Middle Ages when women who were confined to the house retained the tropical dress while men gradually adopted the arctic dress. The history of the costume reflects as in a mirror the social and economic history of Europe. In the feudal society in which every individual was born into a status, every estate had its peculiar costume. Nobility, clergy, members of the professions, artisans and farmers, all dressed differently. Their clothes varied in style and material. The higher the social position, the costlier the materials and the more frilly the dresses. Soldiers had gorgeous uniforms until very recently. Their purpose was to make the soldiers more attractive to the fair sex than other mortals, as a compensation for the professional risks they ran. National costumes of great beauty developed among peasant populations. Some were adaptations of court dresses, others the expression of an innate artistic sense. They have been in use for many centuries with little changes. They are being revived today in many countries as a result of growing nationalism and also because the peasant is more appreciated than in the past.

The rise of the middle class is also accurately reflected in costume. When two worlds clashed in the French Revolution, trousers became a symbol of partisanship. The nobility clung to the breeches, the *culottes,* while the people were *sans-culottes,* that is, they wore not breeches but trousers. The victory of the middle class and the rise of democracy abolished privileged costumes, which were preserved only in the remnants of feudalism, royal courts, the House of Lords, the Catholic Church and similar institutions. When more and more clothing was factory-made and it became possible to produce very attractive dresses for little money, class distinction in clothing vanished almost entirely.

The emancipation of women, the fact that they took an increasing part in the process of production, in sports and other occupations which used to be the exclusive domain of the male sex, had a profound influence on clothing. Matters went so far that women at times even discarded the traditional tropical dress and adopted the arctic mode, wearing pyjamas, slacks and even shorts.

Once clothing was no longer a symbol of class distinction, its sexual function became more pronounced. Since *variatio delectat* in sexual matters too, feminine fashion throughout the democratic era was a constantly shifting endeavor to conceal and reveal the back, breasts, arms, legs and thighs. According to whether women wished to appear feminine or boyish, secondary sexual characteristics were accentuated or minimized. Women in Manet's paintings wear the bustle or *faux-cul*, an ingenious device that put great emphasis on natural rotundities which today are compressed in girdles worn chiefly for the benefit of the silk and rubber industries.

In recent years the development of such a reactionary movement as Fascism has had interesting repercussions on the costume. Since it is a men's movement that would like to relegate women to the kitchen, it has affected only the men's way of dressing. The tendency to regiment the population and to divide it into two main groups, leaders and led, has resulted in the adoption of uniform party shirts. Since Fascism is antidemocratic and hierarchical, it endeavors to clothe as many people as possible in uniforms with insignia of rank, very much as was the case in czarist Russia. The nationalistic trend of Fascism, finally, is responsible for a virtual renaissance of national folk costumes among the peasant population.

We must now try to find out what effect clothing did and does have on health. Ornamental scars, tattoos and similar decorations are not harmful in themselves, but cases are known where the irritation they caused resulted in the development of cancroids and cancers of the skin. Paint can be a protection of the skin but in certain cases also an irritant. All customs of dressing that mutilated or deformed the body obviously had ill effects. The binding of the feet practised for centuries on Chinese girls made them helpless cripples, and the emancipation of Chinese women began with the struggle against this custom. Binding of the feet was never known to the West, but since small feet were considered an attribute of female beauty in many periods, shoes were frequently too small and too narrow, with crippling effect on the toes, so that our ancestors suffered a great deal from corns and ingrown nails. High heels were once worn by upper-class men and women alike. Their purpose was to make the wearer appear taller and to give him a posture and moderate walk that seemed a sign of dignified grandeur. Men discarded high heels with the French Revolution, but women still use them, at least for evening wear, in spite of their inconvenience. Their evil effect is obvious, in that they put the full body weight, not on the whole foot, but on a very small part of it.

The Western world did not bind feet, but for centuries it bound the woman's waist. The corset is a product of the baroque period. Baroque art broke the noble straight line of the Greek pillar and replaced it with the spiral column, developing an architecture of spirals and curves and bulges. The woman's body was subjected to the same laws that determined the style of the period. With a mighty hairdress or wig, a painted face, bulging breasts, a narrow waist and wide skirts made still wider with the advent of the crinoline, woman looked like a flower vase put on a broad pedestal. The French Revolution with its Roman ideals liberated women from the corset, and for two short decades they dressed and looked

24

like Roman ladies. But the Restoration brought back the corset, which then became an unconscious symbol of the still feudal servitude of woman to man. Democracies developed that gave rights to men only. But tens of thousands of women were working—without corsets—in factories. Their labor made possible the development of the textile and many other industries. The time came when they claimed equal rights with men. The corset was thrown aside definitely at about the period when women won the suffrage.

The corset was probably responsible for many of the vapors, faints and fits that befell 18th century ladies. The tighter it was worn, the worse were its effects on health. By compressing the lower part of the chest and the abdominal muscles, it seriously impaired respiration. The corset also deformed the liver, compressing and displacing it as well as the stomach and other abdominal organs; it exerted pressure on the blood vessels so that respiration, digestion and circulation were badly affected. There is hardly a disease that has not been attributed to the corset. This may be an exaggeration, but there can be no doubt that the ill-fated garment had a very bad influence on the general well-being and vigor of women and thus greatly contributed to the development of many cases of illness. If anything, the corset made the fair sex a weak sex.

The human frame has only two places from which clothes may be suspended in a natural way: the hips and the shoulders. It is impossible to attach garments at any other place without using pressure. The Greek and Roman brassiere, the *strophion* or *mamillare*, was a mere double-headed bandage which had to be applied very tightly in order to hold. The present brassiere is far superior in that it is suspended on the shoulders. The mediaeval hose were one piece garments that covered the entire legs and were suspended on the hips. In the 16th century the hose were divided into two parts, stockings and trunk hose, and the attachment of stockings presented a problem that was difficult to solve hygienically. Garters

25

worn below or above the knee had to be tight. Hence they compressed the veins and contributed to the development of varicose veins in individuals having a disposition for such an ailment.

Greek and Roman garments, tunic and cloak, were few, were worn loosely, draped, and were easy to keep clean. From the 13th century on dresses were tailored, materials used were increasingly heavy, and the number of garments worn by an individual increased steadily also. It was more difficult to keep them clean. Dirty clothes are a breeding ground for lice, and lice are the carriers of such diseases as typhus and relapsing fever.

It seems to be a rule that people are the cleaner the fewer clothes they wear. The natives of tropical Africa are very clean. Europe became the filthier the more petticoats and other garments people wore. The new cleanliness is a very recent achievement, despite the fact that in ancient Greece and Rome all classes made frequent use of baths. As recently as 1873 Pettenkofer made the statement that many people were satisfied with one quart of washing water in 24 hours and that bathing facilities were the exception in a Munich household.[17] In those days and even later most people washed their bodies only once a week on Saturday evening or Sunday morning before going to church. And they changed their underwear only once a week. What applied to Germany was true for the whole of continental Europe. England, and America under English influence, were conspicuous exceptions.

The explanation of these conditions is easy to find when we remember that the chief purpose of clothing is decoration. Dirt was never considered an aesthetic sight. Whenever people dressed lightly and exposed much skin, they washed not so much for hygienic as for aesthetic reasons. Clothes, however, covered the dirt and it seemed sufficient to wash the parts that were seen, the face and the hands. A woman's leg clad in silk was attractive, even if it was filthy underneath. A man's shirt that was not seen need not be clean as long as the collar and the cuffs were. These were de-tachable so that they could be changed more often than the shirt.

Cleanliness became the chief postulate of the hygienic move-ment of the 19th and 20th centuries. It had to overcome many obstacles, notably the resistance of people who claimed that the frequent use of soap was harmful to the skin. More serious were religious inhibitions. Christianity, because it related the custom of dressing to the original sin, had overdeveloped the concept of modesty. By insisting that people should cover as much of their bodies as possible, it had endowed nudity with a morbid attractive-ness. Nakedness appeared sinful even in the privacy of the bath-room, and there are still Catholic schools where girls bathe in their shirts. There is no sadder sight than the effect of certain mission-ary activities on the natives of Africa. In Africa pants have become no less a symbol of Christianity than the cross. By forcing the arctic dress on natives of the tropics and imposing a foreign concept of modesty upon them, a conflict has been created that has not im-proved morals and is certainly not in the spirit of true Christianity.

Granted that the chief purpose of clothing is decoration and that it primarily serves to hide or correct physical defects and to heighten the sexual attractiveness of the individual—yet it can-not be denied that in our climates clothing has also an important hygienic function to fulfill. It protects the body against atmos-pheric factors such as cold, rain, or insolation. In order to serve its purpose adequately, it must be so constructed that it does not impede any physiological functions of the body and must consist of materials that are bad conductors of heat in winter, good con-ductors in summer. The porosity of the material, the air content of textiles, is very important in that respect. Great progress has been made in our century. Fashion is, and probably will always be tyrannical, but sports, the fact that more and more women do men's work, and also a growing consciousness of health and enlightenment in health matters have set definite limits to its power. We move in our clothes much more comfortably than our ancestors did.

Inadequacy of clothing in quantity and quality exposes the organism to damage from the atmosphere, and to colds with all their complications. As with nutrition, poverty is the chief cause for inadequate clothing.

One last point must be mentioned in this connection. Civilization developed the custom of covering the body with clothes. Clothing serves health but, as we have seen, can also bring illness. The phenomenon of disease, on the other hand, has also created costumes. In the Middle Ages, for example, the lepers were compelled to wear distinguishing signs so that healthy people would not touch them.

At the time of the Black Death in 1348–1349 some physicians devised a mask and gown to protect them against the contagion. The costume made them an easy target for satire and caricature. Masks, however, proved effective in the plague epidemic that ravaged Manchuria in 1910–1911 and during the epidemic of influenza of 1918–1919.

The rise of asepsis developed a special costume for the surgeon, who now operates clad in sterilized gown and cap, with rubber gloves and a mask in front of mouth and nose to keep germs from the patient. The hospital physician became the "man in white." Orders organized in the Middle Ages for nursing the sick and wounded wore distinctive marks. Thus the Knights Hospitallers of St. John of Jerusalem wore and still wear the eight-pointed cross. In modern time the Red Cross became the symbol of the international organization created by Henri Dunant in 1863. Nursing societies, lay and ecclesiastical, designed costumes for their members.

Paleolithic man sought shelter in caves. The cave was his home; in it he felt safe, protected against the weather and his enemies. Fire provided him with light and warmth, the smoke escaping through the opening of the cave. Drawings sometimes adorned the walls.

As civilization advanced, man no longer had to rely on natural shelters; he built his home. Where the rock was soft he could dig artificial caves and cliff dwellings. The cave could be enlarged by piling up stones in front of it, building walls, covering them with logs or skins. This gave him additional rooms that could be used as granaries, store rooms, or for other purposes.

Tribes living in the forest built round huts by planting sticks in the ground, binding them together at the top and covering them with brush, thatch or skins. A hut was a room. If more rooms were needed, more huts were built just as the natives of Africa still build their kraals.

In the late stone and bronze age rectangular huts were built on piles in the lakes of Central Europe. They were convenient in many respects. Fish could be caught from the platform; refuse could be dumped into the water, and the inhabitants felt well protected. The same type of dwelling is still built in Siam and various parts of Melanesia.

The primitive hut remained for centuries and millennia the shelter of the poor. In Africa and Asia hundreds of millions of people still live in huts which are hardly different from those of the Stone Age. In certain sections of Southern Italy the pre-Roman round hut can still be seen, and in Albaicin, a suburb of Seville, gypsies live like cliff-dwellers in caves dug into the mountain.

When civilization led to the growth of a propertied class a new type of house developed in the ancient Orient. The convenience of having many rooms connected together under one roof suggested the construction of the block house, where many rooms were contained in one block; and of the court house where the rooms opened into an inner court, the *atrium* of the Romans, the *patio* of Spain. These became the prototypes of the house in East and West.

Stone, clay baked by sun or fire into bricks and tiles, timber cut or uncut became the chief building materials. Masonry and carpentry were the crafts that built the houses.

The house is a protection against the weather and thus serves health, but it can also be harmful to health if it does not meet certain requirements. A house must be sufficiently spacious so that the inhabitants have enough air and privacy. This means that a floor area of at least 120 to 150 square feet of living and sleeping rooms should be available per person, not counting kitchen, lavatory, staircase and similar accessories.

Housing suffers from a basic contradiction. A habitation must protect one from the weather, but the air it contains must be renewed constantly if it is not to become vitiated by man's physiological functions and by many of his occupations. The habit of smoking tobacco has greatly contributed to spoiling the atmosphere of the homes. Ventilation is not a problem in warm climates where windows can be kept open the whole year round and people work in the open air, but it is a serious problem in northern regions.

The temperature of a house should be adjusted to the outside temperature so that people can live and work in it without a feeling of discomfort. The simplest method of heating a room was by having a fire in it. The Roman farmer, in winter, had a fire in the center of his hovel, the sparks and smoke escaping through a vent in the roof.[18] The introduction of the chimney was an improvement because it made for better ventilation. The fireplace was the chief heating device in the mediaeval manor and it is still popular in England. As a heating system it is inefficient, but it is a good method of ventilating rooms.

Rooms in Roman city houses were heated chiefly by braziers. They are still used in Southern Europe and in the Orient and represent a most primitive and inadequate heating system. I shall never forget a week I spent working in the library of the Abbey of Monte Cassino in February. When my fingers were frozen stiff I warmed them over a brazier, but the effect never lasted long and I left the place with a severe cold.

The stove originated in ancient Rome when the fireplace was not left open but contained in an apparatus of stone or bricks. In antiquity stoves were used for cooking and baking only. They were used for heating from the early Middle Ages on and were better than open fireplaces because their action was slower and more persistent. Stoves built of so-called Dutch tiles appeared in Switzerland as early as the 9th century. Stoves of cast iron were first used in the 14th century, and the round iron stove became the cheapest and therefore the most popular heating apparatus. Benjamin Franklin constructed a very ingenious stove which made use of the fireplace for ventilation.[19] Iron stoves had the advantage that they developed heat very rapidly but they cooled down just as fast. If the ventilation was not sufficient, the very toxic gas carbon monoxide was produced. Stoves were thus responsible for many casualties. Emile Zola died tragically from carbon monoxide poisoning.

The heating of houses with fireplaces and stoves had the great disadvantage that a room was not warm unless it had its own heating apparatus. Since it was too expensive and too cumbersome to have a stove in every room, only living rooms were heated as a rule. The result was that a house or apartment was heated very unevenly, so that people moving from one room to another were constantly exposed to sudden changes of temperature. Rising in the morning from a warm bed they sometimes had to break the ice before they could wash. Such conditions were certainly not conducive to health. They were responsible for many cases of

31

respiratory diseases, colds and coughs, for lowered general resistance, and to a certain extent for a greater susceptibility to tuberculosis. The primitive hearth and stove also explain why the advent of spring was greeted so exuberantly in former times, being celebrated not only as the ever stirring mystery of the rebirth of nature but also because it relieved man from the many hardships and discomforts of winter.

The introduction of central heating was a long step forward because it made possible a more uniform dispersion of warmth. The Romans are usually credited with the invention of central heating. Archaeological findings have confirmed Vitruvius' descriptions of an ingenious heating system which, however, is totally different from our modern central heating. Air was heated in furnaces and then was conducted into a heat chamber, the *hypocaustum,* located under the floor of a room. It is very likely that hot air also entered the room directly through hollow tiles in the walls. While it comes close to the principle of central heating, yet the hypocaust system was never applied for the heating of entire houses but only of single rooms, particularly of bathrooms.[20] It was still used occasionally in the Middle Ages.

The idea of heating a whole house from one central furnace was conceived in the 18th century.[21] Hot water was used for the purpose in England from 1716 on; hot air was used in the central heating plants of various royal palaces in Russia and Germany in the middle of the century. In 1784 James Watt constructed the first steam heating plant. The system was improved in the early 19th century in England, chiefly by James Perkins. The installation was expensive and for a long time central heating was considered a great luxury. The next step was taken when one central plant was used to heat more than one building. This happened first in 1877, in Lockport, N.Y.

We all know from experience that steam heating has its disadvantages too. Since it is difficult to regulate there is, particularly in American cities, a tendency to overheat buildings and the hot, dry air of many of our apartment houses and offices affects the respiratory organs unfavorably. It may be a contributory factor in the development of our national disease, the "sinus troubles." Nevertheless, too much heat in winter is better than not enough. Since fuel costs money, there are still many people who cannot afford to heat their dwelling places sufficiently and are thus exposed to the injurious effects of the cold.

The artificial cooling of buildings, though extremely desirable, is less important than their heating. In warm climates people sleep during the hot midday hours and are active in the early morning and late evening. In the temperate zone the cold season is long while the hot season is very short. There can be no doubt, however, that modern air conditioning, by lowering the temperature and regulating the moisture of our dwelling places, greatly increases our feeling of comfort and the efficiency of our work. It is in its infancy still and, although the problem may be solved technically, air-conditioning is not yet economically feasible. An air conditioned house is still a luxury available only to a few.

Improvements in the lighting of houses have very deeply influenced man's mode of living. It was the elder Pliny who said that we live as long as we are awake.[22] Thus the electric bulb has actually lengthened our span of conscious life. In the past, as we have seen, the rhythm of man's life closely followed the rhythm of nature. People retired when the sun set and rose with the dawn, as, indeed, the farmers of most countries still do. Throughout antiquity, the Middle Ages and for long thereafter the city people lived very much like the farmers in this respect. Lighting was very primitive in Greece and Rome. Oil lamps gave little light, and were hardly improved until the end of the 18th century when Argand, in Geneva, invented the cylindrical wick. Candles of tallow and wax, made late in antiquity, remained a luxury for many centuries and were used principally in churches and in the houses of the rich.

Lighting was a problem in the daytime also. Glass was made from the middle of the third millennium before Christ, but it was mostly opaque or colored glass, used for vases and other vessels. Windows, both of glass and of mica, have been found in Roman houses but their use was by no means general. Only a few special rooms in rich houses, such as a bathroom that had to be kept tightly closed, were provided with them. When it was cold outside, or very hot, windows were closed with wooden boards or rugs, and the rooms were dark. The Middle Ages produced beautiful stained glass windows, but it took a long time before good transparent glass could be made, and even then only people of means could afford to have many large windows with glass. Several countries therefore imposed taxes on doors and windows, with the result that the poor man's house remained dark and ill-ventilated at a time when cheap glass was easily available.

Poor lighting added to the many hardships that the long winter nights brought upon the people. They probably slept more in the past than they do today. There was no "night life" and no one left the house without necessity or unless he had a sufficient escort. This more sedate life benefited the health of the people, but for those who tried to read or work with insufficient light the cost in eye strain was probably very high.

Conditions changed radically in the course of the 19th century when illuminating gas was introduced. It was applied first for the lighting of streets. In 1808 London had one street with gas lights, in 1814 the whole borough of St. Margaret was supplied with gas, and in the United States Philadelphia had its new lighting system in 1817. Illuminating gas was gradually introduced into the homes. It gave a bright light and was very convenient but, as we all know, not without danger. Gas not only created a new fire hazard but, since it contained carbon monoxide, it was also highly toxic and many casualties resulted from gas poisoning. In the homes it had to compete with a lamp that had been greatly improved by the use of mineral oils. The petroleum lamp had the advantage that it could be carried from one room to another, but it was a fire hazard too. And then, in 1879, Thomas Alva Edison demonstrated the electric bulb which was to inaugurate a new era in lighting.

Today man has conquered darkness and can extend his activities far into the night, adjusting illumination to his needs and to the requirements of every type of occupation. Cities are no longer the gloomy places they used to be after dark. Street lights and neon signs enliven them. People meet in social intercourse, attend shows, work or play at night without ruining their eyesight. Artificial illumination has greatly contributed to the safety of our cities and also to the speeding up of human activities. City people sleep less than they did in the past, often not enough, and so again their health suffers.

Man, as a result of his physiological functions and of his occupations, produces filth. Where many people live close together filth accumulates very rapidly. Filth in itself is not necessarily harmful, but since organic material decomposes it provides a breeding ground for parasites which are a menace to man. Pasteur demonstrated that bacteria occur in greatest number in the immediate vicinity of man. The germs of intestinal diseases are ejected with the stools of patients, which thus become a source of contagion. Sewage and refuse must be removed from dwelling places. Houses must be kept clean. This requires much water and is a tremendous task.

The Romans were fully aware of the hygienic significance of fresh water available in large quantities. Wherever the Romans set foot, we still find the ruins of gigantic aqueducts. As a matter of fact, many of them still fulfill their original purpose. According to Frontinus, in the second century A. D., more than 222 million gallons of water were brought daily to Rome on eight aqueducts. Carcopino and Rowell [23] have shown that little of that water went directly into the private homes and that it had to be carried from public fountains or obtained from water carriers. Water, nevertheless, was available and of good quality.

The Romans also built an elaborate sewerage system that drained the sewage into the Tiber. The mighty arches of the Cloaca Maxima, the chief and oldest sewer, can still be seen. But again it would be a fallacy to assume that every house was connected with the public sewer.

The development of cities in the Middle Ages had ill effects on health. Sanitation was very primitive and water, coming mostly from wells, often had to be carried for long distances. Latrines connected with frequently overflowing cesspools had to be emptied by scavengers. Refuse was thrown into the streets. As a result cities were infested with rats, and from the 14th to the 17th centuries epidemics of plague were frequent and took a heavy toll of lives. Intestinal diseases, typhoid and dysentery, were endemic. The municipal authorities were aware of the danger and from the Middle Ages on measures were taken to improve conditions. In spite of the steady growth of cities, the mortality of the inhabitants continually declined, probably as the result of a rising standard of living. The general yearly death rate of London was 42 per 1,000 of the population in the period from 1681–1690. It dropped to 35 in the 18th century, was 25 in the period from 1846–1855 and is around 12 today. In this decline of the mortality of city dwellers, sanitation, the construction of new water supplies and sewerage systems played an important part. The new public health movement started in England, where great efforts were made from the middle of the 19th century on to improve sanitary conditions. England set an example that was followed by one country after another.

I would like to mention incidentally that the water closet was

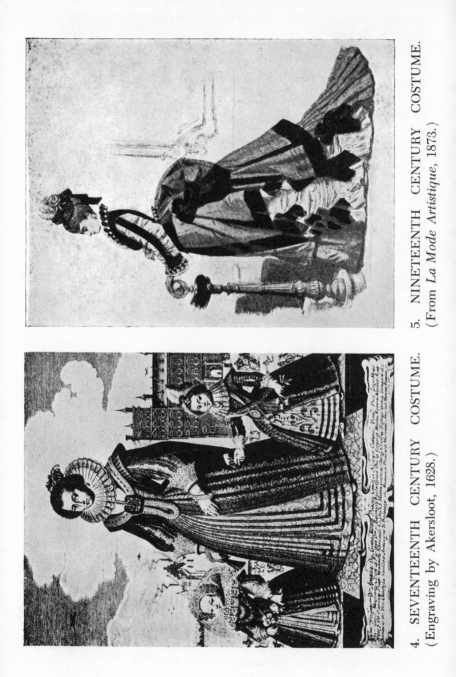

4. SEVENTEENTH CENTURY COSTUME.
(Engraving by Akersloot, 1628.)

5. NINETEENTH CENTURY COSTUME.
(From *La Mode Artistique*, 1873.)

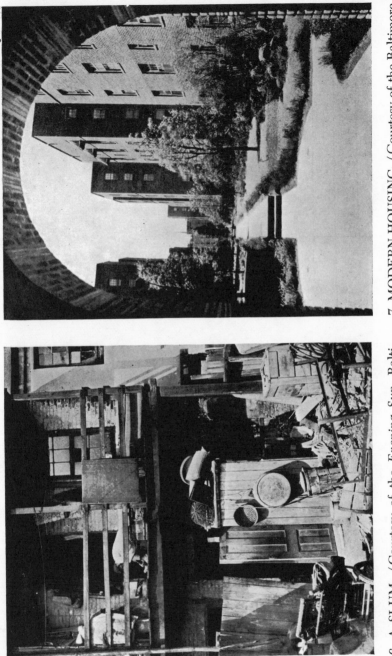

6. A SLUM. (Courtesy of the *Evening Sun*, Baltimore, Md.)

7. MODERN HOUSING. (Courtesy of the Baltimore Museum of Art.)

invented by a poet, a courtier of Queen Elizabeth, Sir John Harington. It was described in an appendix to his *Metamorphosis of Ajax,*
where it appeared under his butler's name. It is said that the
Queen was impressed by the new invention and had it installed
in Richmond Palace, "with a copy of the *Ajax* hanging from the
wall." [24] The water closet was a great hygienic contribution, but it
could not be applied on a large scale before the 19th century, when
the cities built their new water supplies and sewerage systems. At
that time it became almost the symbol of the new public health
movement but it is by no means universally applied even today.

Housing is a difficult problem, particularly in the cities. In the
country the farmer can build a shelter, some kind of a shelter, by
himself, without the help of specialists. The American pioneers
built log cabins in the woods, sod huts on the prairie, which were
later replaced by more permanent buildings. When the home-
stead grew, the farmer added wings to the house, built new barns
and sheds. A well that is used by few people can be kept relatively
clean. Faeces can be buried without too much trouble. Refuse
decomposes on the dunghill with animal excretions and is then
used as manure.

Difficulties begin when people crowd into the cities. Greek and
Roman towns were often built according to plans after sites had
been carefully selected. The mediaeval town developed near the
manor or abbey in a haphazard way. Once it was surrounded by
walls, limits were set to its expansion and houses grew in height.
Many American cities were also built planfully. William Penn's
plan for Philadelphia is well known.

As long as cities grew slowly, plans could be respected. Conditions changed in the 19th century with the rapid development
of industries and in America also with the waves of immigration.
The population increased all over the Western world and masses
of propertyless workers settled in the vicinity of the factories lo-

cated in the suburbs of the cities. In the country the farmer, as a rule, owned his house, but in the city real estate became a commodity, an object of trade and speculation. A house was an investment that could yield high returns. When an industry developed and there was much demand for habitations, the most miserable shacks could be leased for high prices. Slums rapidly developed, in which people were herded together under appalling sanitary conditions. Edwin Chadwick in his classical *Report on the Sanitary Condition of the Labouring Population of Great Britain* of 1842, Frederick Engels in his book *The Condition of the Working Class in England in 1844*,[25] Louis-René Villermé in his *Tableaux de l'État Physique et Moral des Ouvriers Employés dans les Manufactures de Coton, de Laine et de Soie* of 1840, the German Ernst Dronke in his book *Berlin* of 1846,—all these authorities have given a terrifying picture of living conditions in Western Europe towards the middle of the last century.

In American cities conditions were bad enough even before the great industrial development. Speaking of New York, the physician Benjamin McCready wrote in 1837: [26]

> One great source of ill-health among laborers and their families, is the confined and miserable apartments in which they are lodged. In the rapid growth of our city in particular, the number of buildings has by no means increased in a manner corresponding to the great influx of strangers. The accommodations are insufficient, and the rents in consequence extravagantly high. Upon no class of the people does this evil weigh so heavily as upon the laboring population. To give an instance of this—the garret of a small two story building in Catharine-street is divided by board partitions, into three apartments. The stairs leading to the garret are broken and have lost their bannisters, and the flooring of the rooms is broken through in several places. The ceiling in the centre of the garret is not higher than twelve or fourteen feet, and from this it shelves off towards the eaves of the house. For the largest of these rooms, about twelve feet by fourteen, and the only one which has a fire-

place, $1.50 per week is demanded, and for each of the others $1 and $1.25 per week respectively; so that the rent of the garret alone, amounts to $195 per annum. For a cellar, small, damp, lighted by a single broken window, and the walls formed by the naked stones of the foundation through which the moisture was constantly exuding, $65, payable quarterly in *advance*, was demanded and obtained. Nor are these singular examples; in every instance that I have inquired, I have found the rents of the laboring poor in a similar proportion.

Another evil resulting from a crowded population, and the consequent exorbitant rents, is the manner in which houses, intended for the poorer classes of our community, are constructed. In some instances large buildings, designed for breweries or sugar-refineries, have been divided into numerous small, dark rooms, every one of which is tenanted by a family. In other cases the cupidity of landlords has tempted them to build up narrow alleys with small wooden tenements, which, costing but little, and being let to numerous families, yield immense profits. The alley is often not more than six feet wide, paved with round stones and with very insufficient means for draining off the water. It is not uncommon in such situations, to find one or two of the apartments in each house entirely under ground. Can we wonder if in such a state of things we find moral as well as physical disease, vice as well as sickness? Can we expect men who live thus to be sober and orderly, or women to be cleanly and domestic? In such situations, during the summer months, diarrhoea and dysentery are rife, and among children fatal. Scrofula, in some of its protean forms, is frequently met with, and they form the lurking places where small-pox, measles, and scarlet-fever lie covered under the ashes, or when circumstances are favorable, blaze up into sudden fury.

Slums are still the cancer of our cities. The dwelling, meant to protect the peoples' health, has in many cases become a major cause of disease. All our cities, so badly adapted to the present means of transportation and to modern sanitary requirements, need drastic rebuilding. Some progress has been achieved and a few of the worst slums have been demolished, to be replaced by sanitary and pleasant housing developments. The problem, however, is far from being solved, and even people of means who pay high rents often live crowded in their city apartments, with little privacy, disturbed constantly by the neighbors' radios and other savage noises. I am sure that many divorces in the middle class are due to a limited housing space that never really permits the people the simple luxury of "a room of one's own."

If health is vital for human welfare, then housing is certainly an issue of major importance. And if this is the case, housing should not be the object of speculation or source of profit which it is to-day. Competitive business can neither honestly face nor properly solve the housing problem of our contemporary society.

Just as the phenomenon of disease evolved certain costumes, so also it has led to the development of special types of structures. Chief among them is the hospital. In the early centuries of our era, it was a *xenodochium,* a guest house that provided shelter for the indigent and the stranger, and later became a place where the indigent sick were nursed and received free medical treatment. When medical science progressed, giving rise to aseptic surgery and to better diagnostic methods, the hospital was no longer a dreaded place of death, but the center of all medical activities, equally sought by rich and poor.

From the few rooms maintained for the sick in the early me-diaeval monastery, the hospital developed into the stately building with large wards of the late Middle Ages and Renaissance; the pride of a city, as we can still see in the Ospedale Maggiore in Milan. And finally it became the highly complex institution of our days, with sick rooms large and small, solariums, examination and operating rooms, and fully equipped with laboratories and facilities for medical research. The modern hospital has lost the gloom of its precursor, where every feature reminded one of the proximity of death. Today the hospital remains a place of suffering and disease, but the accent is on life.

NOTES

1. See E. Parmalee Prentice, *Hunger and History, the Influence of Hunger on Human History*, New York and London, 1939, a rather uncritical book that must be used very cautiously.

2. Jérôme Carcopino, *Daily Life in Ancient Rome*, ed. by Henry T. Rowell, New Haven, 1940, p. 65.

3. Romesh C. Dutt, *Famines in India*, 1900.

4. W. H. Mallory, *China: Land of Famine*, 1926.

5. See A. Štampar, *Public Health in Jugoslavia*, School of Slavonic and East European Studies in the University of London, 1938.

6. See, for instance, Oribasius, ed. Bussemaker and Daremberg, III, 168 ff.

7. Ludwig Friedländer, *Darstellungen aus der Sittengeschichte Roms in der Zeit von August bis zum Ausgang der Antonine*, 9. Aufl. von Georg Wissowa, Leipzig, 1920, Vol. II, pp. 282–312.—Jérôme Carcopino, *l.c.*, p. 263 ff.

8. Quoted from J. C. Drummond and Anne Wilbraham, *The Englishman's Food, A History of Five Centuries of English Diet*, London, 1939, p. 251.

9. Hugh Bradley, *Such Was Saratoga*, New York, 1940, p. 203.

10. V. M. Molotov, *The Plan and Our Tasks*, Moscow, 1936, p. 63.

11. The Value of Health to a City, translated by Henry E. Sigerist, *Bulletin of the History of Medicine*, 1941, Vol. X, p. 603. Reprinted separately by the Johns Hopkins Press, Baltimore, 1941.

12. *L.c.*, p. 604 f.

13. M. A. van Andel, Der Skorbut als niederländische Volkskrankheit, *Archiv für Geschichte der Medizin*, 1927, Vol. 19, pp. 82–91.

14. *Historische reisen door d'oostersche deelen van Asia*, Amsterdam, 1711, p. 92 ff.

15. Genesis 3, 7 and 21.

16. C. H. Stratz, *Die Frauenkleidung*, Stuttgart, 1900.

17. Max von Pettenkofer, The Value of Health to a City, *l.c.*, p. 607.

18. J. Carcopino, *l.c.*, p. 36.

19. An Account of the New-Invented Pennsylvanian Fire-Places, 1744, reprinted in: Nathan G. Goodman, *The Ingenious Dr. Franklin*, Philadelphia, 1931.

20. Otto Krell, *Altrömische Heizungen*, Munich and Berlin, 1901.—Carcopino, *l.c.*, p. 36 ff.

21. F. M. Feldhaus, *Die Technik der Vorzeit,* Leipzig and Berlin, 1914.
22. *Naturalis Historia,* praefatio 18.
23. *L.c.,* p. 38.
24. See the delightful essay on Sir John Harington by Lytton Strachey in *Portraits and Miniatures,* London, 1931.
25. First published in German in 1845. The first English translation was published in New York in 1886.
26. Benjamin W. McCready, On the Influence of Trades, Professions, and Occupations, in the United States, in the Production of Disease—being the Prize Dissertation for 1837, *Transactions of the Medical Society of the State of New-York,* 1837, Vol. III, p. 97 f.

CHAPTER II

Disease and Economics

IN ORDER to satisfy his wants, man has at all times had to work. Even in tropical regions he had to gather the fruit, to catch the fish and game. Wants increased with every advance in civilization. It was an advantage to be able to grow plants and to raise domesticated animals, because these things gave man increased security; but hard labor was still needed to cultivate and irrigate the soil, to reap the harvest and attend to the cattle. The clothes that adorned and protected the body had to be prepared from skins, or from fibers laboriously woven into textiles. Labor built the hut, made the canoe, hewed stone into tools and lighted the fire. Gradually a primitive division of labor took place: man was the hunter, the cattle breeder and the warrior; woman attended to the fields and to the home.

The growing complexity of civilization was paralleled by a multiplication of wants and an intensification of labor. We sometimes hear that people today spend most of their time working to acquire the means that will permit them to satisfy their wants, while they have hardly any time left for their actual satisfaction. Such a statement is a fallacy in so far as it overlooks the fact that, avowedly or not, the greatest need of civilized man is the performance of creative and socially useful work. This, indeed, is one of the true criteria of civilization: when man is no longer an isolated, self-centered individual, but has become a useful member of a cooperative society.

The farmer's satisfaction is not only that his work feeds him and his family and yields a little surplus with which he can buy a few needed commodities. It is also that he has power over nature; that he is able to increase the fertility of the soil and to direct it. When in the spring the fields are covered with a tender green, and in the summer the heavy ears are ready for the harvest, the farmer is justly proud in the knowledge that this is not only nature's but also his own doing. He loves the good earth, and if his social consciousness is awakened, he also knows that his work upon it is serving one of the basic needs of society. The mechanic who succeeds in repairing a broken-down car feels satisfaction when he hears the first explosion of the motor, not just because it means money for him but because he has tested his skill and found it good.

Indeed, work is not the curse of mankind but its greatest blessing. Work ennobles and gives meaning to our life. It allows us to create those material and cultural values without which life would not be worth living. If society has progressed, it is because of the cooperative efforts of all its members.

Work is a powerful factor in health, balancing our daily life and determining its rhythm. A muscle that is not used becomes atrophied; an inactive brain deteriorates. The unemployed have more than their share of illness not only because of lowered standards of living but also because enforced idleness, by upsetting the rhythm of their lives, has impaired their physical and mental balance.

The evidence of human history has amply demonstrated how human greed and stupidity have brutalized labor so that instead of rewarding us with health it has too frequently penalized us with disease. Work can be harmful in two ways, quantitatively and qualitatively. Excessive labor, not properly compensated by rest and recreation, exhausts body and mind and thus lessens man's natural resistance. On the other hand, there are many occupations that are harmful because the work must be performed under unfavorable environmental conditions.

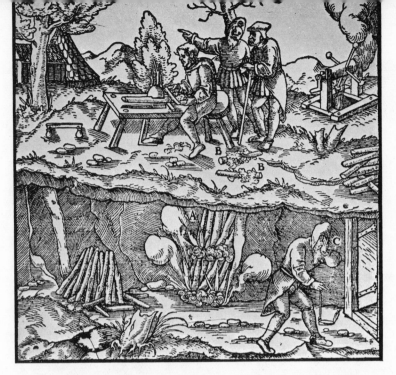

8. HEALTH HAZARDS IN MINES, 17TH CENTURY. (From Georg Agricola, *De re metallica*, 1530.)

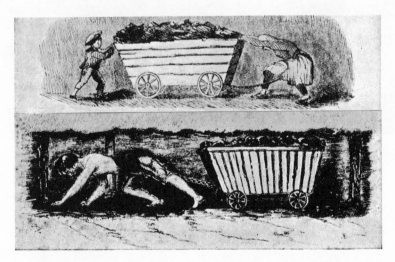

9. LABOR CONDITIONS IN COAL MINES, 19TH CENTURY. (From *Report of the Children's Employment Commission, on Mines and Collieries*, London, 1842.)

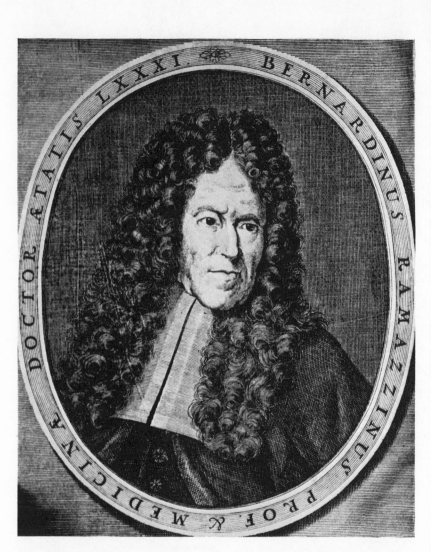

10. BERNARDINO RAMAZZINI (1633–1714). The founder of industrial medicine.

In all ancient civilizations it happened that a small number of individuals appropriated for themselves the land and other means of production. Prisoners of war were made slaves, and ancient economy was largely a slave economy. In disturbed periods, with frequent wars, labor was easily available, and the individual slave's life counted little since he could be replaced without difficulty.[1]

We are inclined to value a civilization in terms of its artistic achievements, many of which have survived the centuries and are as impressive today as in their own times. The Egyptian pyramids reveal a powerful creative spirit and a highly developed technology, but we may too easily overlook the fact that they were built in the blood and suffering of tens of thousands of slaves. We can still see them laboring under the whip as they are represented in Egyptian wall paintings and reliefs. The life of the city worker was not very much easier. An unusual Egyptian document has transmitted to us a voice of rebellion: [2]

> I have never seen a blacksmith acting as ambassador or a foundry worker sent on a mission, but what I have seen is the metal worker at his work: he is grilled at the mouth of the furnace. The mason, exposed to all weathers and all risks, builds without clothing. His arms are worn out with work, his food is mixed up with dirt and rubbish: he bites his nails, for he has no other food. The barber breaks his arm to fill his stomach. The weaver engaged in home work is worse off in the house than the women: doubled up with his knees drawn up to his stomach, he cannot breathe. The laundryman on the quays is the neighbour of crocodiles. The dyeworker stinks of fish spawn: his eyes are tired, his hand works unceasingly and as he spends his time in cutting up rags he has a horror of clothing.

The graceful bronze statuettes of the Greeks still delight us, but we forget that the copper, the tin and the coal needed for making the bronze were mined by slaves and convicts working ten hours a day in narrow galleries, suffocated by heat and smoke.

Ancient industry was mostly on a small scale. Artisans worked frequently in the open air as they still do all over the East. Industrial hazards were, therefore, much less serious than in later centuries. Nevertheless, occupational diseases did occur. A case of lead poisoning is described in the Hippocratic writings,[3] and Pliny speaks of the evil effect of lead, mercury and sulphur on those who handled them.[4] The poets, Martial, Juvenal and Lucretius mention incidentally the dangers of certain occupations and speak of the diseases peculiar to sulphur workers [5] and blacksmiths; [6] of the varicose veins of the augurs [7] and the hard fate of the gold miners.[8] Nothing was done to protect them unless they helped themselves, as did those minium refiners who, according to Pliny,[9] put membranes and bladder skins, as masks before their faces. Medical service was provided only for those who served to entertain the people, the gladiators.

Towards the end of the Middle Ages and in the Renaissance the demand for metals increased considerably. The development of trade called for more gold as a medium of exchange. Firearms which were increasingly used after the 14th century required large quantities of lead, copper and iron, and thus greater supplies of raw materials for the developing industries. Many shallow mineral deposits were exhausted and people were forced to dig deeper into the soil. The deeper the mines, the more hazardous mining became. Danger threatened from water, gases and mechanical injuries. It is not an accident that the first monographs on occupational diseases of miners were written in the 16th century. Paracelsus who had acquired a great deal of practical experience in mines inaugurated this type of literature. His book *Von der Bergsucht und andern Bergkrankheiten,*[10] written probably around 1533–1534 and first published in 1567, was the first of a long series of books on that subject. Beginning with Agricola's *De re metallica,*[11] published in 1556, every book on mining had a chapter on the diseases of miners.

Mining was the basic industry of this period, and also the most dangerous. Other industries were less harmful, but each had its peculiar hazards. The goldsmiths were exposed to fumes and smoke; for them Ulrich Ellenbog, a German physician in Augsburg, wrote as early as 1473 a small pamphlet *Von den gifftigen besen tempffen und reuchen* [12] that circulated in workshops in manuscript form and was finally printed around 1524.

Health conditions and health hazards in industry and in various occupations before the industrial revolution are splendidly illustrated in Bernardino Ramazzini's great classic on occupational diseases, *De morbis artificum diatribe,* first published in 1700.[13] Again it is not an accident that such a book was written at just that time. The 17th century was a mechanical age, and many of its notable physicians were *iatromechanists.* Ramazzini himself says that "nowadays medicine has been almost entirely converted into a mechanical art, and in the schools they chatter continually about automatism." [14] Physicians who constantly compared organs with tools could not but be interested in workmen's tools and machines.

A chance observation drew Ramazzini's attention to the subject: [15]

> I will relate the incident that first gave me the idea of writing this treatise on the diseases of workers. In this city, which for its size is thickly populated, the houses are naturally close together and of great height, and it is the custom to take the houses one by one every three years and clean out the sewers that run in every direction through the streets. While this work was going on at my house I watched one of these workmen carrying on his task in that cave of Charon and saw that he looked very apprehensive and was straining every nerve. I pitied him at that filthy work and asked him why he was working so strenuously and why he did not take it more quietly so as to avoid the fatigue that follows overexertion. The poor wretch lifted his eyes from the cavern, gazed at me, and said: "No one who has not tried it can imagine what it costs to stay more than four hours in this place; it is the

same thing as being struck blind." Later, when he had come up from the cesspit, I examined his eyes carefully and observed that they were extremely bloodshot and dim. I asked whether cleaners of privies regularly used any particular remedy for this trouble. "Only this," he replied, "they go back at once to their homes as I shall do presently, shut themselves in a dark room, stay there for a day and bathe their eyes now and then with lukewarm water; by this means they are able to relieve the pain somewhat." Then I asked him: Had they a burning sensation in the throat or any respiratory troubles or attacks of headache? Did that stench hurt their nostrils or cause nausea? "Nothing of that sort," he replied, "in this work our eyes only are injured and no other part. If I consented to go on with it any longer I should very soon become blind, as has happened to others." Thereupon he wished me good-day and went home, keeping his hands over his eyes. After that I saw several workers of this class with eyes half-blinded or stone-blind begging alms in the town.

Ramazzini examined the working conditions and health hazards of forty-one vocations, discussing the diseases peculiar to them, their treatment and prevention. He added a dissertation on *Diseases of Learned Men,* and for the second edition he wrote a supplement of twelve chapters describing conditions prevailing in a dozen other crafts. His distinction between two great groups of occupational diseases, one based on the material used and one on the labor involved, was very good indeed and was accepted by most physicians who wrote on the subject thereafter. Very modestly Ramazzini considered his book an "imperfect performance," but it soon became authoritative, was reprinted several times, translated into various languages, and little was added to the subject until the industrial revolution created new conditions.

In America the literature on occupational diseases began in 1837 with a prize essay written for the Medical Society of the State of New York by Benjamin McCready.[16] The American economy was still primarily agricultural, and McCready raised the

48

question quite seriously whether it would not be better for the country to remain agricultural instead of developing industries. At that time the great canals and the first railroads were being built. New England had textile mills driven chiefly by water power, but otherwise industry was still in its handicraft stage. The conditions pictured by McCready, therefore, are not very different from those described by Ramazzini. McCready attributed the ill health of many workers not so much to the occupation itself as to the general working and living conditions, poor ventilation of shops, poor housing, filth, lack of exercise in many occupations, and intemperance. On some public works laborers received a daily allowance of five glasses of whisky as part of their wages.

In an interesting passage which deserves to be quoted in full, McCready thinks that much of the ill health of the American people is due to their striving after wealth:

> The population of the United States is beyond that of other countries, an anxious one. All classes are either striving after wealth, or endeavoring to keep up its appearance. From the principle of imitation which is implanted in all of us, sharpened perhaps by the existing equality of conditions, the poor follow as closely as they are able the habits and manner of living of the rich. From the lower prices of provisions, and from the cheaper rates of house rent, families could formerly be supported much more comfortably and abundantly, on the same means, than they can be at present; and the artizan compares the ease which he formerly enjoyed with his present condition. Every one has seen immense fortunes made in a short time by successful speculation, and a rage for such speculation has infected all classes of the community. From these causes, and perhaps from the nature of our political institutions, and the effects arising from them, we are an anxious, care-worn people. Now, however favorable this may be to our industry and enterprize, it cannot but be deleterious to health. How far these injurious effects may extend, it is impossible to determine; but we may observe that when causes act thus gen-

erally, however trifling their consequences may seem with respect to individuals, when they regard the mass, they cannot fail to be very considerable; and when we reflect that in all probability every deterioration of the general health of the parents is transmitted to their offspring, the subject becomes one of great importance. For my own part I have little doubt that the pale and unhealthy appearance of our population, is in a measure owing to the very causes which have contributed to the rapid rise and unexampled prosperity of our country.

The industrial revolution in the beginning affected the people's health very adversely. The new industries created employment for large numbers of unskilled workers including women and children. The population of Europe increased and large numbers of immigrants began to crowd in the suburbs of American cities. They worked long hours under appalling hygienic conditions. They lived in slums, without sanitation, on minimum standards and every economic crisis subjected these socially useful masses to still greater pauperism and still more dependence on charity for survival.

Conditions became so bad that society was stirred. It was justly felt that a sick working class was a menace to the health of all. A very fine little book published in 1831 by a physician in Leeds, C. Turner Thackrah, on *The Effects of the Principal Arts, Trades, and Professions, and of Civic States and Habits of Living, on Health and Longevity,* revealed striking figures. In the industrial city of Leeds in 1821 there was one death for every 55 inhabitants, while in a neighboring rural district there was one death per 74 inhabitants. "At least 450 persons die annually in the borough of Leeds, from the injurious effects of manufactories, the crowded state of population, and the consequent bad habits of life," was the conclusion of Thackrah who then proceeds (second edition, 1832):

Every day we see sacrificed to the artificial state of society one and sometimes two victims, whom the destinies of nature would have spared. The destruction of 450 persons year by year in the borough of Leeds cannot be considered by any benevolent mind as an insignificant affair. Still less can the impaired health, the lingering ailments, the premature decay, mental and corporeal, of nine-tenths of the survivors, be a subject of indifference. Nor is it in Leeds only that inquiry produces so painful a result. Leaving out of the question London and the Seaports, we might prove that Sheffield, Manchester, Birmingham, in fact, all our great manufacturing towns, exhibit an equal or a greater excess of mortality,— and an excess increasing with the magnitude of the population. If we should suppose that 50,000 persons die annually in Great Britain from the effects of manufactures, civic states, and the intemperance connected with these states and occupations, our estimate I am convinced would be considerably below the truth. Can we view with apathy such a superfluous mortality, such a waste of human life? Assuredly an examination of our civic states and employments has long been demanded, alike by humanity and by science.

Thackrah wrote his courageous book "to excite the public attention to the subject." He was well aware that the upper class did not like to have this subject discussed but he was convinced that conditions could be, and must be, improved:

Most persons, who reflect on the subject, will be inclined to admit that our employments are in a considerable degree injurious to health, but they believe, or profess to believe, that the evils cannot be counteracted, and urge that an investigation of such evils can produce only pain and discontent. From a reference to fact and observation I reply, that in many of our occupations, the injurious agents might be immediately removed or diminished. Evils are suffered to exist, even where the means of correction are known and easily applied. Thoughtlessness or apathy is the only obstacle to success. But even where no adequate remedy immediately presents itself, observation and discussion will rarely fail to

51

find one. We might even say, that the human mind cannot be fairly and perseveringly applied to a subject of this kind, without decided effect.

Thackrah's findings were more than confirmed by the monumental *Report on the Sanitary Condition of the Labouring Population of Great Britain* published by Edwin Chadwick in 1842. And the Asiatic cholera which from 1831 on swept in repeated epidemics over Europe was a convincing argument, for it played havoc with the working population and was threat to all.

Improvements were made, but very slowly. The English "Health and Morals of Apprentices Act" of 1802 limited the laboring hours of children in cotton mills to twelve. The Act of 1833 forbade the employment of children under 12 years of age for more than 8 hours a day, of children of from 13 to 18 years for more than 12 hours. Factory inspectors were appointed as enforcement officers, but nevertheless there were many abuses. In 1842 the employment of women and of children under 10 years to work underground was forbidden. The 10-hour working day for women and children was introduced in 1847, but children under 10 years of age were permitted to work in English factories until 1874.

Sanitary conditions improved after the Public Health Act of 1848 had inaugurated a series of public works. The right of the workers to organize labor unions was recognized in England in 1824–1825. In a struggle of over a century they succeeded in gradually improving their working and living conditions.

England was the first country to experience the full impact of industrialization, which did not fully mature in continental Europe and the United States until later. Conditions varied but every country sooner or later was forced to protect its workers through labor laws.

Today in most Western countries we live in industrialized societies. Commodities are produced in factories in large quantities, and even agriculture has become increasingly technical and mechanized. Whether or not we like this development makes no difference; we must accept it as a fact. There is no return to the handicraft industry of the Middle Ages. Modern machine industry has come to stay; it has raised the standard of living considerably, and has thus greatly contributed to the well-being and health of the people. On the other hand, there can be no doubt that industrial work has created many new health hazards. The laborer is in constant touch with physical or chemical forces of high potency. Furthermore, as a result of the extreme division of labor, work has become monotonous and it is difficult for the worker to realize that he is taking part in a creative process of great importance.

The wealth of nations is produced primarily by the labor of the industrial and agricultural workers, and the least that society can do is to reduce their hazards by all available means. It must always be kept in mind that the purpose of the machine is to promote human welfare, a purpose which is obviously defeated when labor becomes harmful. The protection of labor requires scientific research, the establishment of standards, and legislation to enforce them. Industrial accidents and diseases are a responsibility of the employer who must attend to them without delay or cost to the worker, and with proper compensation for the loss of wages and for disability. The first industrial clinics were opened in 1910, in New York and in Milan. Workmen's compensation was first introduced into Germany in 1883 as part of a general social insurance scheme. The first British compensation law was passed in 1897. When it was revised in 1906 thirty-one industrial diseases were included. America, with its highly developed industry, was one of the last countries to introduce workmen's accident compensation. Laws were passed from 1900 on and are in force today in all but one state. There are, however, still many states that do not compensate for industrial diseases.

Many occupations that society needs are harmful to health, even under the best possible hygienic conditions. The only way to counteract their evil effect is by reducing working hours and by providing paid vacations for rest and recreation. Vacations, as a matter of fact, are not enough. The coal miner who inhales dust the whole year round, the steel worker who constantly handles the white-hot metal, the girl in the textile mill who works standing at the loom, the fruit picker after a season of back-breaking labor, —all need more than an annual vacation. They are in want of medical repair. We overhaul our machines regularly and know that it is more economical to have minor repairs made before they break down completely. Why should we not apply the same principle to human conservation? A sound program of preventive medicine must foresee not only annual vacations for the working population and means of rest and recreation; it must also provide periodic examinations and all facilities required for the treatment of minor ailments before they develop into serious diseases.

The growth of industry would have been impossible without the cooperation of women. Their labor virtually created the textile industry, and eventually has contributed more than anything else to their social and economic emancipation. Once firmly established in the process of production, with incomes of their own, women were entitled to claim equal rights with men. Women, however, always carry an additional physiological burden of immense social significance, the bearing of children. Society, therefore, must make special provisions for the protection of the health of working women. It must exclude them from particularly harmful or physically strenuous occupations, must grant them paid leaves before and after delivery, must provide nurseries for the children and effect other protective measures.

Industrialization has radically changed the social structure throughout the world. A hundred years ago in most Western countries the majority of gainfully employed persons consisted of independent producers; today the great majority are wage earners and salaried employees who depend for a living on the labor market. The insecurity of capitalist production is a factor that affects the people's living standards and thus their health very deeply. They have accepted the duty to work and may justly claim it as a right. Steady employment under the best possible hygienic conditions, the correct balance between work, rest and recreation, and wages that permit a decent standard of living—these are basic and significant factors of public health.

In any given society the incidence of illness is largely determined by economic factors, some of which have already been mentioned in the previous chapter. A low living standard, lack of food, clothing and fuel, poor housing conditions and other symptoms of poverty, have always been major causes of disease.

Health conditions have greatly improved, at least in the Western world, but this improvement has not equally benefited the various groups of the population. The process was in many cases as follows: a disease, such as tuberculosis or malaria, indiscriminately attacked all groups. With developing civilization the standard of living rose and medicine advanced. Groups in the higher income brackets were the first to profit from these gains, leaving the disease to continue its ravages among the people of low income. A few examples may illustrate this economic determination of illness.

The decrease in the mortality from tuberculosis has been stupendous. The annual tuberculosis death-rate for every 100,000 population was around 450 in Massachusetts in 1857. It dropped steadily and reached 35.6 in 1938. It was 190.5 in the United States in 1900 and 48.9 in 1938. These, however, are average figures. When we analyze them, we soon find significant variations in the different social groups. A few generations ago the disease occurred in all classes. Today it is primarily associated with low income groups, and especially with the unskilled laborer and his family. That is why in America the negro carries a much heavier load of tuberculosis than the white man.

An analysis of the incidence of tuberculosis in the various districts of the city of Paris, in France, revealed that in 1923–1926 the average death-rate was 130 in the well-to-do 16th district while it was 340 in the 20th, a working class district.[17] The variations within this one city were even more striking in 1926, when the 8th district had a death-rate of 75 and the 13th one of 306. This was a ratio of one to four, or about the same as existed in the incidence of tuberculosis among whites and negroes in the United States. In 1924 a group of 17 blocks in Paris with 4,290 houses and a population of 185,000 had a death-rate of 480. In other words, the mortality was higher there in 1924 than it was in Massachusetts in 1857.

American statistics of Rollo H. Britten published in 1934 [18] illustrate very graphically the rôle of economic determination in disease. The mortality from pulmonary tuberculosis per 100,000 for the age groups from 25 to 44 years in 10 states was:

Professionals	28.6
Clerks	67.6
Skilled workers	69.0
Unskilled workers	193.5

This applies not only to tuberculosis but to other diseases also, although the differences are not so outstanding. According to the same study, the percentage of deaths due to pneumonia was:

Professionals	5.8
Clerks	6.5
Skilled workers	7.2
Unskilled workers	9.4

The uneven distribution of disease reflects itself also in the general death-rate, the annual number of deaths per 1,000 population. At a time when it averaged 8.7 for all gainfully employed, it was:

Professionals	7.0
Clerks	7.4
Skilled workers	8.1
Unskilled workers	13.1

A survey by Sydenstricker, Wheeler and Goldberger of *Disabling Sickness among the Population of Seven Cotton Mill Villages of South Carolina in Relation to Family Income* [19] showed the following relation between half-month family income per adult male and case rates of sickness prevalent in May–June, 1916, per 1,000 persons canvassed:

Under $6	70.1
$6–7.99	48.2
$8–9.99	34.4
$10 or over	18.5

We sometimes hear that the high incidence of illness in low income groups is caused not so much by economic factors as by lack of stamina and by poor hereditary endowment in the people involved. These, we are told, are responsible for both the low economic status and the high incidence of illness. The *Health and Depression Studies* carried out by the U. S. Public Health Service during the recent economic crisis discredit such a thesis.[20] A survey was made to determine the disability rates of 12,000 wage-earning families, including 49,000 individuals who had suffered from the depression in varying degrees of severity. House to house canvasses were made in 8 large cities and 2 representative groups of smaller communities. Complete data were assembled on these families for the four-year period from 1929 to 1933. Their median income was $1,650 in 1929 and $870 in 1932. The results were extremely interesting. They can be summarized in the following points:

1. The rate of disabling illness was 48 per cent. higher in fam-

ilies with no employed member in 1932 than in families having fully employed members.

2. The families that dropped from fairly comfortable circumstances to relief status showed a rate of disabling illness 73 per cent. higher than that of families which remained in comfortable circumstances during the four years.

3. The families that dropped from comfortable to moderate circumstances showed a rate of disabling illness that was 10 per cent. higher than that of families remaining in comfortable circumstances.

4. The families that dropped from moderate to poor circumstances had a rate of disabling illness 17 per cent. higher than that of families remaining in moderate conditions.

5. The rate of disabling illness in families that dropped from comfortable to poor circumstances was 9 per cent. higher than that of families that had always been poor.

All the evidence we have points to a very close relationship between the economic status of a population and the volume of illness which it carries. Even the most advanced countries have in their low income groups a large reservoir of disease.

A next step in the development is taken when a country succeeds in overcoming a disease entirely. In such a case the disease is, so to say, outlawed from the country but it continues to exist elsewhere, chiefly in the economically backward lands. This has happened with many communicable diseases.

Plague, which ceased to be a problem to the Western world from the 18th century on, still exists in Asia and Africa. The epidemic that broke out in Asia in 1896 did not reach Europe. From 1903 to 1921 ten million people were killed by the plague in India alone. Even such a highly infectious disease affects the various socioeconomic groups differently. In one of the Indian epidemics the deaths per 1,000,000 population were: [21]

Low cast Hindus	53.7	Jews	5.2
Brahmins	20.7	Parsees	4.6
Mohammedans	13.7	Europeans	0.8
Eurasians	6.1		

Many other communicable diseases, such as cholera, yellow fever, and typhus, were in a similar way driven out of the economically advanced countries, but we are by no means rid of them. We continue to breed them in backward countries where at any time they can become a menace to us. A war, a revolution, any event that upsets the very subtle machinery of public health control, can lead to the violent resurgence of an epidemic that may spread without any regard for political boundaries. The last world war gave rise to epidemics such as the world had not seen since the Middle Ages. And today, in the winter of 1941–1942, typhus is already beginning to flare up on the eastern front.

The conclusions to be drawn from these facts are obvious. In every country disease must be attacked with all available means and where it is most prevalent, in the low income groups. And since the world has become very small as a result of the present means of communication, we must think and plan not merely on a national but on an international scale. There is a human solidarity in health matters that cannot be disregarded with impunity. Today, in spite of all medical progress, more than one billion people, chiefly in Asia and Africa, live under health conditions that are as bad as the worst the Western world ever experienced in the course of its history. Our task is therefore by no means solved. It calls not just for medical, but even more for wide-spread social and economic measures. Thus, the problem of public health is ultimately political.

One more aspect of our problem must be discussed in this chapter, namely, the economic consequences of disease.

Illness not only creates suffering but is also an economic loss. The sick man cannot work and therefore loses his wages. Illness frequently disables a man permanently or for a long time. He becomes unemployable, and the result may be that a whole family drops in the social scale. Thus illness generates poverty, which in turn generates more illness. The economic hazards of sickness, however, reach beyond the sick man and his immediate dependents into society as a whole in that the latter is deprived of the diseased citizen's labor power, temporarily or permanently. In addition, tens of thousands of individuals die in every country prematurely, without necessity, from maladies that could have been prevented or cured. Every such case of premature death is a capital loss to the nation. Disease thus interferes directly with the economic life of society by destroying labor power and the means of subsistence of individuals and groups. The loss is increased when society has to provide funds to care for the victims of illness; a large percentage of all relief money is spent for the support of people who have become indigent as a result of illness.

Many diseases can be prevented and many can be cured. But prevention and cure cost money. Society must provide a living for physicians, public health officers, dentists, nurses, and other medical personnel. All of these must be trained in costly institutions and large sums of money must be expended on research to increase the knowledge that permits them to act effectively. The hospital, which is playing an increasingly important part in all aspects of medical care, has also raised its costs considerably. Finally, medical supplies, such as drugs and appliances, are needed in rapidly growing quantities.

Some medical care is obtainable collectively through public, charitable, or philanthropic funds, but most of it must be purchased by the individual, and usually at a time when he is financially handicapped by illness. The risk of sickness, though unpredictable for the individual, can be estimated accurately for large groups. In order to spread the risk among a number of people, as well as to pool their resources, the principle of voluntary insurance has been applied, from the mutual benefit funds of mediaeval guilds to modern consumers' health cooperatives. Compulsory health insurance for wage-earners and salaried employees was introduced in Germany in 1883 and thereafter in a great many other Western countries. Medical care was made a public service financed through taxation in the rural districts of Russia in 1864, and the Soviet Union has "socialized" all medical services.

No one could realize the tremendous extent of economic losses caused by illness until figures were made available for certain communities or countries. In a pioneering effort, Max von Pettenkofer in 1873 set out to estimate the value of health to his home city of Munich.[22] Munich in those days had a population of 170,000 and the very high general death-rate of 33 per 1,000. In other words 5,610 people died in the city every year. Pettenkofer had good evidence for assuming that the average annual number of days of sickness was 20 per capita of the population so that the total loss of time amounted to 3,400,000 days. Estimating the average loss of money caused by the loss of wages and the costs of medical care at 1 florin [23] a day—a very conservative estimate—it became apparent that the population was losing every year 3,400,000 florins on account of illness, an enormous amount in those days. Sickness was levying a toll of 5 per cent. on the people's working time. These were impressive figures even without the inclusion of capital losses due to premature death.

Pettenkofer then calculated how much the city of Munich would save if it succeeded in reducing its death-rate from 33 to 22, which was then the mortality rate of London. He showed that this would save every year 1,870 human lives, 63,580 cases of illness and 1,271,600 sickness days. This meant a saving to the people of 1,271,600 florins. Capitalized at 5 per cent., such an amount would represent 25,432,000 florins. The wealth of Munich would be increased by that much merely as a result of improved health conditions.

Sixty years later, in the United States, the Committee on the Costs of Medical Care found that the country in 1929 had spent 3.6 billion dollars for medical care, classified as follows:

		(in million dollars)
I. *Personnel*		
	1. Physician	1,090
	2. Dentist	445
	3. Nurse	
	(a) Graduate	142
	(b) Practical	60
	4. Secondary personnel	
	(a) Midwife	3
	(b) Optometrist	50
	(c) Chiropodist	15
	5. Sectarian Practitioner	125
	Total Cost of Personnel	1,930
II. *Hospital*		
	Operation of hospital	656
	Capital construction	200
III. *Private Laboratories*		3
IV. *Commodities*		
	1. Drugs	665
	2. Glasses	50
	3. Orthopedic appliances	2
V. *Public Health*		121
VI. *Various Organized Services*		29
	Total Cost of Medical Care	3,656

The economic loss caused by illness, of course, amounts to much more than 3.6 billion dollars. To the costs of medical care must be added the loss of wages and the capital loss due to premature deaths. It has been estimated on good grounds that the people of

the United States lose ten billion dollars every year as a result of illness.[24]

NOTES

1. See H. E. Sigerist, Historical Background of Industrial and Occupational Diseases. *Bulletin of the New York Academy of Medicine,* 1936, 2nd Series, Vol. 12, pp. 597–609.

2. Papyrus Sallier, 2, 4, 6, and f.

3. Epid. IV, 25; ed. Littré V, 164–166.

4. Nat. Hist. XXXIV, 50; XXXIII, 40.

5. Martial, Epig. XII, 57, 14.

6. Juvenal, Sat. X, 130.

7. Juvenal, Sat. VI, 397.

8. Lucretius VI, 811.

9. Nat. Hist. XXXIII, 40.

10. *On the Miners' Sickness and Other Miners' Diseases.* Translated from the German, with an Introduction by George Rosen. In: *Four Treatises of Theophrastus von Hohenheim Called Paracelsus,* edited, with a preface by Henry E. Sigerist, Baltimore, The Johns Hopkins Press, 1941, pp. 43–126.

11. An English translation by H. C. Hoover and L. H. Hoover was published in London in 1912.

12. *On the poisonous wicked fumes and smokes.* A facsimile of the German original was published by Franz Koelsch and Friedrich Zoepfl in Munich, 1927.

13. A first English edition was published in 1705 under the title: *A treatise of the diseases of tradesmen, shewing the various influence of particular trades upon the state of health; with the best methods to avoid or correct it, the useful hints proper to be minded in regulating the cure of all diseases incident to tradesmen.* A new edition of the Latin text of 1713, revised, with translation and notes by Wilmer Cave Wright was published in 1940, University of Chicago Press.

14. Ed. Wright, p. 11.

15. *L.c.,* pp. 97, 99.

16. On the Influence of Trades, Professions, and Occupations, in the United States, in the Production of Disease, *Transactions of the Medical Society of the State of New York,* 1836–1837, vol. 3, pp. 91–150; new edition by Genevieve Miller, in preparation.

17. These and the following figures from R. Pierreville, *L'inégalité humaine devant la mort et la maladie,* Paris, 1936.

18. *Public Health Reports,* 1934, Vol. 49, pp. 1101–1111.

19. *Public Health Reports,* 1918, Vol. 33, pp. 2038–2051.

20. G. St. J. Perrott and Selwyn D. Collins, Relation of Sickness to Income and Income Change in 10 Surveyed Communities. *Public Health Reports,* 1935, Vol. 50, pp. 595–622.

21. Victor C. Vaughan, *Epidemiology and Public Health,* St. Louis, 1923, Vol. II, p. 781.

22. *The Value of Health to a City,* Two Lectures Delivered in 1873 by Max von Pettenkofer. Translated from the German, with an Introduction by Henry E. Sigerist. Baltimore, The Johns Hopkins Press, 1941.

23. The exchange value of a florin or gulden was about 40 cents at that time but its purchasing power was much greater.

24. I. S. Falk, *Security Against Sickness,* New York, 1936.

CHAPTER III

Disease and Social Life

NOBODY lives alone. Even the most destitute individual who has neither relatives nor friends is a member of a group, a member of society, endowed with obligations toward it and endowed with rights. We live in a highly specialized society which can make good use of every degree of intelligence, skill and strength. The charwoman who keeps my office clean, the letter carrier who brings our mail, can do their jobs well without possessing unusual intelligence and training. Yet our work would be impossible without theirs which is socially useful and entitles them to receive in exchange the means for leading a decent and healthy life.

The ideal cooperative society would be one in which each individual would hold the position for which he is best fitted, in which he would contribute to the general welfare according to his ability, and from which he would receive according to his needs. Such a society seems Utopian today because it presupposes an educational standard, general and political, that we have not yet reached. It also presupposes an economy of plenty that we do not yet possess. Civilization, however, is still very immature and there is no reason why the development from the competitive to the cooperative society should not take place—perhaps sooner than we expect.

As we have seen, when a man falls ill he ceases to be a useful member of society. He drops out, so to say, and may even become

a burden to his fellow men. The more differentiated a society becomes, the more it is affected by the ill health of its members. In a cooperative society, however, useful jobs can be provided even for the physically handicapped. It is interesting to see what great efforts the Soviet Union has made to keep the partly disabled individual at work and by all available means to prevent the skilled worker from dropping into the ranks of the unskilled laborer on account of illness. I have seen blind people performing skilled work in many factories, and other plants have special workshops for the physically handicapped where the speed of the conveyor belt is adjusted to their capacity. Cripples are organized in craftsmen's cooperatives. All this is very uneconomical from our point of view because the productivity of such individuals is obviously reduced below the normal. It is only possible in a society which is itself the employer. In a competitive society the ever so slightly disabled worker cannot keep up with the worker in full health, and thus may easily become permanently unemployable.

The goal of medicine is not merely to cure diseases; it is rather to keep men adjusted to their environment as useful members of society, or to readjust them when illness has taken hold of them. The task is not fulfilled simply by a physical restoration but must be continued until the individual has again found his place in society, his old place if possible, or if necessary a new one. This is why medicine is basically a social science.

The attitude of society toward the sick man and its valuation of health and disease have changed a great deal in the course of history. At all times disease isolated its victims socially because their lives are different from those of healthy people. The sick man is thrown out of gear with life, finds himself confined in his movements, is helpless and compelled to rely on the assistance of others.

The present position of the sick man in society is very complex,

the result of historical developments that we must analyze briefly if we are to obtain a clear view of the subject.[1]

There are very few truly primitive tribes left in the world. Among them the Kubu in Sumatra seem to merit close study, in the opinion of van Dongen, Hagen, Volz and other anthropologists who have investigated them very carefully.[2] The Kubu live in the primeval forest. Minor diseases, skin eruptions, wounds and similar ailments are frequent with them. People suffering from such diseases are not considered different from other tribesmen, for their criterion is social, not physical. As long as a man is able to live the life of the tribe, his condition does not cause any reaction on the part of the individual or of society.

Things are different in the case of serious diseases, more especially those involving fever such as an epidemic of smallpox invading the region, an event which happens not infrequently. Such a patient finds himself unable to take his part in the life of the tribe; he is incapacitated, and there is a sharp reaction which leads to his abandonment both by the tribe and by his own kin. All avoid him as they would a corpse, making his isolation complete. The sufferer is dead socially long before physical death has overtaken him.

The Kubu does not inquire into the cause of disease, which he accepts as he accepts rain or thunder, without any explanation. In the case of tribes living in a higher state of civilization, however, we find a very pronounced desire to ascertain the cause of disease. The sick man is considered a victim, unable to live like other people because someone has worked upon him. An enemy has done something to him, has bewitched him by introducing a foreign object into his body through magic, or else by depriving him of something necessary for his life; or again, it was a spirit or a demon that afflicted him, that entered into him and took possession of his body. Thus the sick man enjoys a special position in society, claiming the regard of his fellow men as well as their help. He is the guiltless victim of secret powers which are recognized and warded off by the medicine man.

If we proceed to a still higher stage and examine conditions in the Semitic civilizations of the ancient Orient, we encounter the opinion that the sick man is by no means an innocent victim but is rather one who through pain is making atonement for his sins. Disease then becomes a punishment for sin. We encounter this view in Babylonia, and it is clearly expressed in the Old Testament. God, we are told, has revealed his law: all who follow it in piety will live in happiness, but those who transgress it will be punished. Disease and suffering are inflicted by way of chastisement, in retribution for the sins of the individual, of his parents, or even of his clan. This was a concept of pitiless logic and of the clearest simplicity. In view of so implacable a doctrine, a figure such as that of the righteous Job suffering unrighteously was all the more tragic.

Where such a view prevailed, the sick man found himself burdened with a certain amount of odium. He suffered, but it was believed that he suffered deservedly. His disease proclaimed his sin for all to see. He was branded, and socially isolated in a particularly severe way. Disease, however, was not only a punishment; it was also an atonement for guilt, and thus a redemption.

The position of the sick man in the classical age of Greek society was quite different. The Greek world was a world of the healthy and sound. To the Greek of the 5th century B. C. and long thereafter health appeared as the highest good. Disease, therefore, was a great curse. The ideal man was the harmonious being, perfectly balanced in body and soul, noble and beautiful. Disease, by removing him from this plane of perfection, made of him an inferior being. The sick man, the cripple and the weakling could expect consideration from society only so long as their condition was capable of improvement. The most practical course to take with a weakling was to destroy him, and this was done frequently enough.

The ancients knew nothing of an organized care of cripples; the diseased or disabled man had to recover if he were ever to count again as a full-fledged being. The physician helped him to reach this end, and since the goal, health, was valued so highly the physician was among the most highly esteemed of the craftsmen. If, however, the patient's condition was hopeless, his malady incurable, medical treatment seemed senseless both for physician and patient, since the end in view was unattainable. The Greek physician would have considered it unethical to attend a hopeless case.

Thus the sick man in Greek society also found himself burdened with an odium, not that of sin but of inferiority.

It remained for Christianity to introduce the most revolutionary and decisive change in the attitude of society toward the sick. Christianity came into the world as the religion of healing, as the joyful Gospel of the Redeemer and of Redemption. It addressed itself to the disinherited, to the sick and afflicted and promised them healing, a restoration both spiritual and physical. Had not Christ himself performed cures? Disease is no disgrace, is not a punishment for the sin of the sufferer or of others, nor does it render the patient inferior. On the contrary, suffering means purification and becomes grace. Illness is suffering and suffering perfects the sufferer; it is a friend of the soul, develops spiritual capacities and directs the gaze towards the Infinite. Disease thus becomes a cross which the patient carries in the footsteps of his Master.

The grace of suffering can be shared by the healthy through sympathy for—suffering with—those who are diseased. "I was sick and ye visited Me. Inasmuch as ye have done this unto one of the least of these My brethren, ye did it unto Me." It became the duty of the Christian to attend to the sick and poor of the community. Through the rite of baptism a man became a member of the Christian family, with all the duties and privileges that a child has in its home. And when Christianity became the official religion of

69

the state, the family embraced the whole of society, and from then on society assumed the obligation to care for its sick members.

The social position of the sick man thus became fundamentally different from what it had been before. He assumed a preferential position which has been his ever since. The care of the sick was organized on a community basis in the beginning of our era and has been continued through the centuries. The motivation has varied in the course of time: in the early centuries it was Christian charity becoming to a large extent humanitarianism in the 18th and 19th centuries. Today we care for the indigent sick for practical reasons also, realizing that society is seriously handicapped by having sick members and that diseased groups are a menace to the whole population.

The attitudes of society towards the sick that prevailed before the Christian era were never entirely overcome. In the Middle Ages and the Renaissance epidemics were very frequently considered visitations inflicted by God upon mankind. Until very recently there were still people who considered mental diseases a punishment for a disorderly life and venereal diseases a singularly appropriate chastisement because they manifested themselves in the organs with which people had sinned. The old retributive view of disease is also expressed in the outraged feelings of patients who consider their sufferings as undeserved.

The sick man, because of his preferential position, finds himself released from many duties. The sick child is automatically excused from school, the sick adult is not expected to work and is exempted from many obligations which society claims from its healthy members as a matter of course. We shall discuss in the next chapter how legal procedures have been revolutionized by the concept of limited responsibility.

The more pronounced the preferential position of the sick became, the more obvious was the inclination to escape from the struggle of life and to take refuge in the condition of illness. This is at the bottom of the condition commonly called hysteria, as Eugen Bleuler has pointed out.[3] The hysterical individual evades the unpleasant reality by suddenly becoming deaf, or blind, or lame with no apparent organic lesion. Hysteria is a disease of which no normal individual would avail himself as a mechanism of escape. The same is, to a certain extent, true of malingering. Whoever evades duties by pretending, or producing, or protracting an illness does it primarily in order to acquire the preferential position granted to the sick man, but he does it on a basis of a pathological condition. Malingering is not a normal psychological mechanism, at least not under ordinary circumstances.

Disease, all forms of disease, invariably affect the individual's social life. So far, we have discussed the general social consequences of illness: we must now consider briefly the influence of some special diseases on the sick man's position in the social structure.

No disease has ever had more dire consequences for the patient's life than *leprosy*. This is a chronic affliction which develops very slowly, the person affected living with it for many decades before he finally succumbs. Leprosy is not very contagious, much less so than tuberculosis, and its contagiousness alone could not explain why society reacted so violently against it. There must be other reasons. Chief among them is probably the fact that the disease mutilates its victims in a horrible manner: one member after another rots away, and this, combined with the evil smell that develops from the gangrenous parts, makes the leper in advanced stages a terrifying sight. Society always reacts very strongly to the physical appearance of a sick man. The emaciated body of a tubercular patient calls forth nothing but feelings of compassion, while skin diseases are considered disgusting. A relatively harmless skin

71

affection can render an individual unemployable and mere pimples can poison a girl's social life. A skin disease reveals to everybody that a system is sick, while many much more serious conditions may remain hidden to the superficial observer. An aggravating factor in the case of leprosy was that the disease was known to be incurable.

Leprosy is a disease of the tropics, where it still prevails. It invaded Western Europe in the early Middle Ages, was endemic particularly among the poor, and reached its peak in the 14th century, declining sharply thereafter. The disease then gradually died out in Europe with the exception of a few spots in the East and North of the continent.

When leprosy in the early Middle Ages began to be a menace to society, the people reacted vigorously against it. Since no physical cure was known and the physicians were helpless, the only way to attack the disease was by social means. So the church undertook to combat it. This was done by applying precepts of Leviticus. The crucial passages found in chapter 13 were the following:

1. And the Lord spake unto Moses and Aaron, saying,
2. When a man shall have in the skin of his flesh a rising, a scab, or bright spot, and it be in the skin of his flesh like the plague of leprosy; then he shall be brought unto Aaron the priest, or unto one of his sons the priests:
3. And the priest shall look on the plague in the skin of the flesh: and when the hair in the plague is turned white, and the plague in sight be deeper than the skin of his flesh, it is a plague of leprosy: and the priest shall look on him, and pronounce him unclean.
45. And the leper in whom the plague is, his clothes shall be rent, and his head bare, and he shall put a covering upon his upper lip, and shall cry, Unclean, unclean.
46. All the days wherein the plague shall be in him he shall be defiled; he is unclean: he shall dwell alone; without the camp shall his habitation be.

The same rules were applied in the Middle Ages. Segregation of the lepers for life seemed the only measure available for the protection of society. Individuals suspected of suffering from the disease had to be reported to the authorities. They were examined, and since the diagnosis had such terrible social consequences the examination took place under particularly solemn circumstances, never being carried out by one physician alone but by a group of doctors who shared the responsibility. In Italy a lawyer was frequently added to the group because the diagnosis had legal consequences. Physicians and patient were under oath. The doctors were exhorted to proceed with great care [4] and to remember well the symptoms of true leprosy, to ponder over them repeatedly, and not to trust a single symptom but only a combination of them, to differentiate between characteristic and non-characteristic symptoms, and to be careful in formulating a judgment. It was explained to the patient that the disease meant the salvation of his soul, and that Christ had not despised such sick persons although human society ostracized them.

If the diagnosis was uncertain, the sick were temporarily segregated *in loco remoto a toto populo* and were later re-examined. But when the diagnosis was established beyond any doubt, the leper was segregated for life. He was expelled from human society and deprived of his civic rights; in some places a Requiem was held for him, and thus he was declared dead as far as society was concerned. He lived in a *leprosarium* outside the city walls in the company of other lepers, all of whom were dependent on charity for their sustenance. In the city of Treves he was given the following instructions: [5]

> You shall never enter the churches, the market, the mill, the bakery, nor attend any meetings.
>
> You shall never wash your hands or whatever you may wish to wash in springs, and when you wish to drink, you shall dip the water with your cup or some other such vessel.

Wherever you go, you shall wear your leper's coat so that you may be recognized by others and you shall never walk outside of your house barefoot.

Whatever you may wish to buy you shall not touch except with a rod.

You shall not enter any inn or other house and when you buy wine, pour it into your flask.

You shall not have intercourse with any woman not even with your own wife.

If somebody encounters you on your way and asks you a question, do not answer before you have moved aside from the direction in which the wind is blowing.

If you pass a bridge, do not touch the rail before you have put on your gloves.

You shall not touch children or any other young people nor shall you give them anything that belongs to you.

You shall not eat or drink in the company of other people but with lepers alone, and you shall know that when you shall have died you will not be buried in the church.

Patients suffering from leprosy are very susceptible to secondary infections. When the Black Death ravaged the world in 1348 and 1349, killing off one quarter of the entire European population, the lepers were the first to succumb to the plague. Many leprosaria were closed after 1349 for lack of inmates, and from then on the disease rapidly declined.

Today lepers are still segregated wherever Christianity is the dominating religion. Society is not afraid of tuberculosis but is terrified by leprosy, chiefly on account of the Biblical tradition. There is no medical indication for segregation, which, on the contrary, may even be harmful because families are inclined to hide a sick member so as not to lose him. In doing so they deprive the patient of medical treatment and supervision. In Japan and other non-Christian countries lepers are treated but not segregated, with the same results as in countries that segregate.

There are economic reasons for segregation. The majority of lepers are indigents and it is cheaper and more effective to keep them together in a leprosarium than to treat them individually in their homes or to have them run around as beggars. In the leprosarium, moreover, they live with fellow patients and escape the social ostracism that would inevitably befall them as soon as the disease reached an advanced stage. Many modern institutions are very well equipped with educational and recreational facilities. As a result of improved treatment many cases are arrested and the patients are released on parole. This makes all the difference in the world. Segregation in a leprosarium is no longer a verdict for life as it used to be; there is still hope for the patient. Besides, many countries are not rigid in their regulations. If the economic status of a patient makes it possible for him to maintain a certain standard of hygiene, he is left free, although he stays under medical supervision. Leprosy, nevertheless, still is one of the great curses of mankind and of all diseases the one that has the most serious social consequences.

The attitude of society towards sufferers from *venereal diseases* has also changed a great deal in the past centuries, and in a very characteristic way. I cannot discuss the origin of syphilis in Europe because I do not know what it was. It is possible that the disease occurred during the Middle Ages without being recognized as an entity of its own, but it is also very possible that it was imported from the New World; the question is still highly controversial and far from settled.[6] At any rate, syphilis was clearly recognized at the end of the 15th century in Europe, was wide-spread, and presented much more acute symptoms than it does today. It was considered a new disease and was described and discussed in a rapidly increasing number of publications.[7]

In the beginning, the venereal source of infection was not clearly understood.[8] The disease was accepted as a catastrophe, like other epidemics. Some attributed its origin to natural factors, to swampy exhalations, or to cosmic factors, to a special configuration of the planets; others looked upon it as a divine punishment. The people had indulged in ungodliness and blasphemy, and God was punishing them by sending this disease among them, as he had sent other plagues before. The malady was believed to spread in epidemic fashion, and every country attributed it to its neighbor. There was no stigma attached to syphilis and great efforts were made to combat it. Towards the end of the 15th century the city of Frankfort provided free medical treatment to syphilitics and as a special inducement made them tax-exempt for the period of their cure. Since the disease had cutaneous symptoms, it largely fell into the realm of the surgeons, who treated it with mercury. They applied massive doses of mercurial ointment, and the treatment, although efficacious, was considered a torture in itself.

In the decade from 1520 to 1530 the sexual character of the infection was generally recognized, and from then on the attitude towards the disease was largely determined by the general attitude towards sex. As long as extra-marital relations were not condemned by society, the disease was taken as a very unpleasant accident, to be sure, but one that did not involve any moral reprobation. The Renaissance was very tolerant in sex matters; brothels were generally accepted institutions and nobody thought of concealing the fact that he had been contaminated. Emperors and kings, noblemen, lay and ecclesiastical, scholars and poets were known to be suffering from syphilis. The humanist Ulrich von Hutten wrote, in elegant Latin, a book in which he described his own case in great detail.[9] He wanted others to benefit from his experience. He had suffered atrociously, not only from the disease but also from the mercurial treatment, and was full of praise for a new remedy that was being imported from America, the guaiac wood. The chief importers, the Fuggers in Augsburg, eagerly promoted the theory of the American origin of syphilis, for it seemed obvious that an

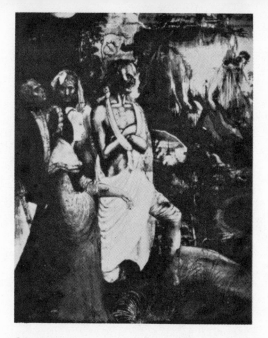

11. BEGINNING AND END STAGES OF LEPROSY. (From a painting by Nicolaus Manuel Deutsch, early 16th century. Basle Museum.)

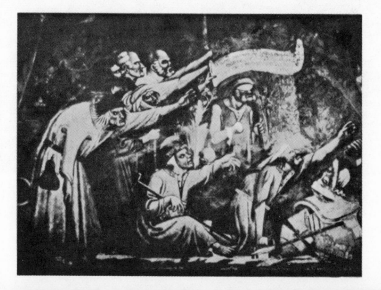

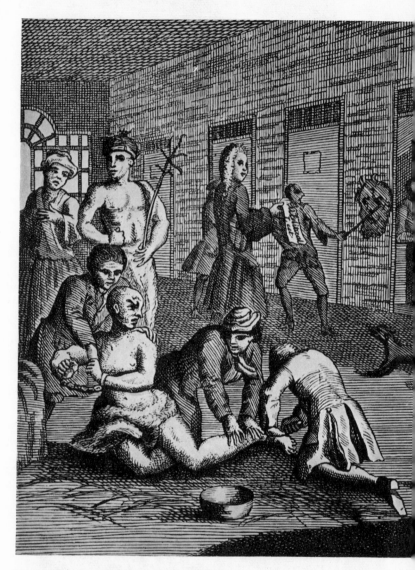

13. WARD IN BETHLEHEM HOSPITAL ABOUT 1745. (From D. H. Tuke, *Chapters in the History of the Insane in the British Isles*, London, 1882.)

American disease could best be cured by a drug that came from overseas. Guaiac was the favorite remedy of the physicians who had also become interested in the new disease. The treatment by inunction was a dirty and brutal method, good for surgeons who treated the common people but not for learned doctors. The Renaissance had a very sober, matter-of-fact attitude towards syphilis, which it considered a painful affliction, but not basically different from other diseases. The venereal patient was neither better nor worse than other men.

The attitude of the upper classes towards syphilis became decidedly frivolous in the *siècle galant*. The symptoms were apparently less acute and the treatment was improved when mercury was given in pills. In a century of great sexual licentiousness syphilis was taken as an unavoidable little accident. It was the cavalier's disease, the wounds caused by the darts of Venus which Mercury, however, cured. Jokes were made and little songs were written about it.

Conditions changed radically with the rise of the middle class. A new attitude toward syphilis developed in the course of the 18th century, to become dominant in the 19th century. The middle class from its very beginning condemned sexual licentiousness and emphasized the sanctity of the family. Virtue, or at least the appearance of it, was demanded from its members. By adopting such an attitude the bourgeoisie claimed to be better than the nobility and therefore entitled to power. But it also endeavored to compensate for the ruthlessness of the economic system that it was constructing on the ruins of feudalism.

Venereal diseases are usually acquired in extra-marital intercourse. The victim, therefore, was marked as a licentious individual, as one who had broken the rules. He was disgraced, and his family keenly felt the stigma. Syphilis and gonorrhoea were not ordinary diseases. They were shameful, not to be mentioned aloud, and certainly not in good society. The young man who after a spree found himself contaminated hid his illness; if he had not the money to seek proper medical treatment, he went to a quack rather than ask his father for help. Convention forbade inquiring after a young man's health before marriage, and many young women were infected by their husbands whose gonorrhoeas flared up during the honeymoon.

In religious circles the view that venereal diseases were an appropriate punishment for sin was wide-spread. In 1826 Pope Leo XII banned the use of the condom because it defied the intentions of divine Providence, namely, to punish sinners by striking them in the member with which they had sinned.[10] And even in the beginning of our century there were church people who were deeply disturbed by Ehrlich's discovery of salvarsan.

Where such views prevailed, the venereal patient had a very special position in society, and one that made it extremely difficult for medicine to combat these diseases. Middle class countries in which the puritanical tradition is strong, even today have not yet entirely overcome this attitude, as we know well enough in America. As a result, they have a much higher incidence of venereal diseases than other countries in which a new and healthier attitude has evolved.

This new attitude developed out of a growing social consciousness. The venereal diseases were recognized as a menace not merely to the individual but to society at large; as a plague that undermined the vitality of individual and nation alike. They struck indiscriminately at "guilty and innocent"—in the United States 60,000 children are born every year with the handicap of congenital syphilis. In a number of countries society took notice of the threat and called upon the state power for protection: Denmark, the Soviet Union and Germany are among those that have enacted strict laws with the purpose of eradicating venereal diseases. Treatment is free but compulsory and whoever evades it commits an offense and is punishable by law. Still more guilty is the individual who spreads the disease by infecting another person: according to the German law of 1927 he can be jailed for three years. In all countries where this attitude has developed venereal diseases are rapidly disappearing. Will this affect the morals of the people, as many fear? The answer is obvious: when a nation has reached a high degree of social consciousness and is strongly aware of its social responsibilities, it does not require the aid of disease to preserve the morals of its people.

Leprosy has virtually disappeared from the Western countries of the temperate zone. The venereal diseases are receding rapidly in the socially advanced countries, and the day is not so far distant when *tuberculosis* will also be a disease of the past. Three factors are responsible for the incidence of tuberculosis: the bacillus that Robert Koch discovered in 1882, the hereditary disposition of individuals, and their social environment. As we mentioned in a previous chapter, the decrease in the incidence of tuberculosis has been considerable in the last fifty years, and there can be no doubt that this was primarily the result of improved social conditions.[11]

The influence of tuberculosis on the lives of those afflicted with it is variously determined. It is not an awe-inspiring disease like leprosy, nor was any moral condemnation ever attached to it as with the venereal diseases. More than any other sick person, the tubercular patient was considered a tragic figure, especially as the disease attacks with preference people in the prime of life. It is essentially chronic and as a rule develops slowly. The mental faculties of the patient remain unimpaired and are perhaps even stimulated by the slightly increased temperature. The sex urge is stimulated also, whether by the temperature or by some factor in the chemistry of the disease, we do not know. Even while they languish and cough their way towards death, the tubercular are full of hope and are always making plans for their future life.

It is a well known fact that many men and women of genius

suffered from tuberculosis.[12] It would be absurd to assume that the disease gave them their creative power. Where there is no genius, no disease in the world can provide it. On the other hand, there can be no doubt that to suffer from tuberculosis is a profound experience which must reflect itself in the work of a creative artist. We shall examine this problem in more detail in a later chapter.

The sanatorium treatment of tuberculosis has brought a new note into the sociology of the patient. In the sanatorium the sick man lives in a somewhat unreal atmosphere. He has been removed from his normal environment and finds himself transplanted into totally new surroundings, located usually amid beautiful landscapes, in the woods or in the mountains. Here he is neither expected nor allowed to work, and he has no obligations towards society, being cared for, nursed, well nourished, and as a rule living on a much higher standard than ordinarily. In other words, he is to a very high degree granted the privileged position of the sick man. If he is a medically indigent person, he lives in the sanatorium as the guest of society, which thus manifests interest in him and wants him to recover. In many cases an entire family has contributed every cent available to make it possible for its sick member to obtain the treatment. The patient, by the mere fact of his condition, has become a person of some importance. His fellow patients are all suffering from the same disease, and this gives the tuberculosis sanatorium an atmosphere that is quite different from that of a general hospital.

The patient has only one task, namely, to recover. Recovery is the goal and purpose of his being in a sanatorium. He wishes to live, to be healthy again and return to his family. Unconsciously, however, he feels that the moment he recovers he will lose his privileged position, will no longer be important, at least not in the same sense, and will have to resume the drudgery of everyday life. With this comes a very conscious fear of the future: will the recovery last? will he find a job? The doctors recommend light work in the open air: but is there such a job and will it permit him to support his family decently?

All this sometimes creates a resistance with which the physician must reckon. His task is not only the physical restoration of the patient; he must also prepare him psychologically for the process of readjustment and assist him in it. Tuberculosis is an extremely social disease and the best medical treatment is simply wasted if it is not combined with social measures. There is no point in curing a patient only to send him back to the slums; the after-care is just as important as the sanatorium treatment, which is but one link in a chain of social measures that begins with education and early case-finding and ends with social rehabilitation.

The Papworth Village in England, a settlement where patients are not only treated but rehabilitated, where they can live with their families and work in various industries as useful members of society, has amply demonstrated what can be done even within the present social structure, and it is only to be regretted that there are not many more such institutions.

The history of those suffering from a *mental disease* is a sad chapter in the medical history of society. It is sad because for many centuries mentally sick persons were treated abominably, and because, of all medical disciplines, psychiatry is still the most backward. In the United States 50 per cent. of all hospital beds—more than half a million—are filled with mental patients, and many thousands are outside of institutions merely because there are not enough accommodations available. No other diseased group requires such an enormous amount of hospitalization, and this proves unmistakably that medicine is still very helpless in the case of most mental diseases.

Psychology, like other scientific disciplines, has progressed. We know today much more about the workings of the normal and diseased mind than we did fifty years ago, and it is possible to keep in adjustment with their surroundings many neurotic individuals who in the past would have remained hopelessly intractable. As regards psychoses, however, we are still impotent, unless we are dealing with those varieties that are the result of infections or intoxications. There is evidence to show that psychoses may often develop on the basis of some hereditary disposition, and where this is so we can do little to cure them.

Mental diseases very profoundly affect the social life of those afflicted with them. Mental patients are conspicuously different from normal people. They perceive, feel, think, act, and react differently; this isolates them, sometimes very severely. The catatonic patient can live for a long time motionless in complete detachment from the world.

There are no sharp borderlines between sanity and insanity. Most mental patients appear physically as normal, and this naturally affected the attitude of society towards them. Medicine was concerned primarily with physical ailments, and a man who looked normal but acted irrationally did not necessarily attract the attention of the physician. On the contrary, it seemed much more logical to assign him to the priest, the physician of the soul. It is much to the credit of Greek medicine that it recognized insanity as a disease condition which did concern the physician, although many mental patients undoubtedly sought treatment in the temples. Harmless ones were left to the care of their families or must have roamed the streets as beggars as they still do in the Orient. Many must have perished for lack of care.

Greek psychiatry survived in the Middle Ages and is reflected in the works of medical writers. In a period, however, that was dominated by religion, the religious approach to insanity was necessarily strong. A man who talked and acted differently from other people appeared as one who was possessed by an evil spirit, by a demon. The cure then consisted in driving out the spirit through exorcism and other procedures. Christ had done so and had given his disciples the same power. All the paraphernalia of primitive medicine were applied in Christianized form in the treatment of the insane.[13]

Possession by a demon was in itself an accident and not a crime. Christ had not punished demoniacs but had cured them by driving out the evil spirit. With the belief in witchcraft, however, it was assumed that witches had been seduced by the devil or had entered into a pact with him: they had become infidels and their crime was heresy. As heretics they were not treated but punished. The penalty was death at the stake. The *Malleus Maleficarum,* the Witches' Hammer, was published in 1489, and in the following centuries thousands of mentally sick persons suffered torture and death *ad maiorem Dei gloriam.*

While the blows of the witches' hammer were falling heavily, some philosophers and physicians—but not many—took a different attitude towards the insane.[14] In the 16th century the Spaniard Juan Luis Vives, a great humanist, psychologist and social reformer, looked upon the insane as sick people who needed gentle treatment. The physician Paracelsus, without denying the existence of witches, considered mental diseases as spiritual in nature, and Johann Weyer in his book *De Praestigiis Daemonum* (1563) took an open stand against witch-hunting. Keenly interested in mental diseases, he recognized that the women persecuted as witches were definitely sick in mind and in need of medical treatment.

Witches continued to be burned at the stake, although in decreasing numbers, until the end of the 18th century. The rise of rationalism helped to overcome an attitude which in itself was a persecution mania. But even the treatment of those patients who were not victimized was bad enough. If they had no family to attend them or if they were violent and a menace to their community, they were confined to poorhouses, almshouses, or to jails where many lived for years chained to the walls like wild animals and whipped by brutal guardians. Special asylums for the confinement of insane persons had been founded from the end of the Middle Ages in various countries,[15] but they hardly differed from prisons.

Under the influence of the humanitarian movement society gradually awoke to its responsibility towards the mentally ill. The chains were stricken from them dramatically during the French Revolution when Philippe Pinel liberated his patients at the asylum Bicêtre in Paris. In England the Quakers pioneered in this humanitarian effort as in so many others: upon the recommendation of a merchant, William Tuke, they founded the York Retreat in 1796 where patients were treated kindly.

In the 19th century the chains fell in one country after another, but frequently they were merely replaced by strait-jackets. It was long before we had learned the lesson that violence is no cure for violence. Brutal treatments still occur sporadically in backward institutions, but they are condemned by society, which no longer considers that mental patients are just "crazy," objects of hilarity when they are harmless, of scorn when violent. The vocabulary has changed. The noxious words "insane" and "asylum" are avoided. Science has shown that mental diseases are not the result of illicit passions but rather their cause. Mental patients are, at long last, generally recognized for what they are: sick people in need of rational medical treatment, and when such treatment fails, deserving humane care.

We can readily assume that in antiquity a great many feeble-minded individuals perished for lack of attention before they had reached the age of reproduction. We mentioned earlier that it was a regular policy in Sparta to expose weak and crippled infants. All this contributed to an elimination of those who were considered to be unfit or poorly equipped by nature for the struggle to survive. Other attitudes developed under the influence of religious views. Thus, in India the belief in the transmigration of souls and the Buddhist postulate of universal compassion resulted in the preservation of every living being, man and animal. In the West, the Christian belief in the immortality of the soul; the view that the purpose of life was salvation; the concept of charity and later, that of humanitarianism—all these ideas had similar results. As a consequence, every nation is today carrying a heavy burden of individuals many of whom are disabled by hereditary diseases and disease conditions, and who will never be able to perform any function in our present society, sometimes living without even being conscious of it. Germany in the last ten years has embarked on a vast sterilization program, in order to prevent the reproduction of the dysgenic. It is a socio-biological experiment that deserves to be watched carefully, even if the present Nazi regime has made it subservient to a thoroughly reactionary—and unscientific—politico-racial ideology.

NOTES

1. See H. E. Sigerist, Die Sonderstellung des Kranken, *Kyklos,* 1929, Vol. 2, pp. 11–20, and *Man and Medicine,* New York, 1932, chapter II.

2. A. W. Nieuwenhuis, Die Anfänge der Medizin unter den niedrigst entwickelten Völkern und ihre psychologische Bedeutung, *Janus,* 1924, Vol. 28, p. 42 ff.

3. E. Bleuler, *Lehrbuch der Psychiatrie,* Berlin, 1916, p. 378 ff.

4. For this and the following see *Examen Leprosorum* in Conrad Gesner, Scriptores de chirurgia optimi, Zurich, 1555, fol. 391 b.

5. O. Schell, Zur Geschichte des Aussatzes am Niederrhein, *Archiv für Geschichte der Medizin,* 1910, Vol. III, pp. 335–346.

6. G. Sticker, Entwurf einer Geschichte der ansteckenden Geschlechtskrankheiten, *Handbuch der Haut- und Geschlechtskrankheiten,* Bd. 23, Berlin, 1931.— E. Jeanselme, Histoire de la Syphilis, *Traité de la Syphilis,* Vol. I, Paris, 1931.

7. Karl Sudhoff, The earliest printed literature on syphilis, Florence, 1925, *Monumenta medica,* Vol. III.

8. For this and the following see the very illuminating study of O. Temkin, Zur Geschichte von "Moral und Syphilis," *Archiv für Geschichte der Medizin,* 1927, Vol. XIX, pp. 331–348.

9. *De guaiaci medicina et morbo Gallico liber unus,* Mainz, 1519.

10. G. Vorberg, *Zur Geschichte der persönlichen Syphilisverhütung,* Munich, 1911, p. 21.

11. See the excellent study of Georg Wolff, Tuberculosis and Civilization, *Human Biology,* 1938, Vol. 10, pp. 106–123, 251–284.

12. Lewis J. Moorman, *Tuberculosis and Genius,* Chicago, 1940.

13. See e. g. the treatment *ad demoniosos* in: H. E. Sigerist, The Sphere of Life and Death in early mediaeval manuscripts, *Bulletin of the History of Medicine,* 1942, Vol. XI, pp. 292–303.

14. See Gregory Zilboorg, *A History of Medical Psychology,* New York, 1941.

15. See George W. Henry, Mental Hospitals, in Zilboorg, *l.c.,* pp. 558–589.

CHAPTER IV

Disease and the Law

IT MAY seem far-fetched to look for relationships between disease and the law, and yet there can be no doubt that they exist and that they have manifested themselves in various ways in the course of history. I know little about jurisprudence and this chapter will appear very amateurish. However, I should like to sketch a few lines of development if for no other reason than to stimulate research in an interesting field that has been very much neglected in the past.

There never has been any form of social life without some form of social control. Individuals living together, be it as a family, clan, tribe or nation, had to observe certain rules of conduct. There is social life among animals also, and it also follows definite rules which, however, are merely instinctive patterns. As long as man lived like an animal in the forest, his rules of conduct were of the same kind as those of other higher animals. With developing civilization, however, the relationships between man and man, and between man and the objects of his environment became increasingly complicated and called for laws to prevent and solve social conflicts. Prohibitions and commandments regulated man's life. Laws were enforced and transgressions punished by whoever had authority over the group; the mother, the father, the shaman or the chief. It was a long way from the religious taboos of primitive people to the *Corpus Iuris Civilis* of Justinian, the way from a primitive to a highly developed civilization, but the ends to be attained were very similar nevertheless.

We saw in the preceding chapter that disease gravely disturbs social life. The individual by becoming sick suffers harm himself and may often inflict harm upon others. Not only does society lose his labor power, but in the case of contagious diseases the sick become a direct menace to the health of their fellow men. Hence society, endeavoring to protect itself, made its sick members the immediate object of legislation.

Many primitive people had a very clear concept of the contagiousness of certain diseases, and taboos were applied to those afflicted with them similar to the taboos applied to the dead. In all ancient cults impurity or uncleanliness was considered a contagious condition: whoever touched an "unclean" person became unclean himself and was not admitted to the temple without having undergone purification rites. Uncleanliness was the result of physiological processes such as menstruation, childbirth, and death, and also of pathological conditions. The leper was unclean, but according to Leviticus so was also the man who had a discharge from the urethra. His bed, his saddle, "every thing whereon he sitteth" was considered unclean.[1] He was to be kept out of the camp.[2]

We have seen that the regulations of Leviticus were applied on a large scale in the Middle Ages in the combating of leprosy. When the Black Death, bubonic and pneumonic plague, invaded the Western world in the 14th century and caused terrific ravages, legislation was enacted to ward off the plague; these old mediaeval regulations are still the foundation of many of our modern epidemiological measures. Patients believed or found to have the disease had to be reported to the authorities, and the number of reportable diseases increased from century to century. Such diseases are no longer considered a private matter of the individual; they are a public concern since the community is menaced by them. Houses in which such patients live are today marked as they were in the Middle Ages in order to warn the citizens. The treatment of such patients is a protective measure in the interest of society. Plague-ridden patients were treated by municipal physicians in the Middle Ages; today in most civilized countries contagious patients are treated free of charge in public hospitals irrespective of their financial status. When a patient died, the plague house was disinfected. This was done in a rather crude way in the Middle Ages. Clothing and bedding were burned; furniture was washed thoroughly with soap and exposed to the sun; rooms were fumigated. Today we know the bacteria that cause such diseases, and we have more effective chemical and physical methods of destroying them, but the underlying idea is the same.

Plague invaded a community from outside. Hence in times of epidemics the cities kept their gates closed and carefully guarded the surrounding highways. Nobody was admitted before he had been questioned and examined very carefully. In-coming mail was fumigated and coins and other objects were dipped into vinegar. It was well known that plague had its origin in the East, whence it spread along the highways and particularly along the sea lanes. The chief danger spots, therefore, were the port cities. On July 27, 1377, the city council of Ragusa ordered that all travelers coming from plague-ridden countries should be barred from the city unless they had spent one month on the island Mercana *ad purgandum*. Venice followed the example and segregated overseas travelers on the island San Lazzaro. The period was eventually extended from thirty to forty days: hence the name *quarantine* originated for one of the most important epidemiological measures that arose in the Middle Ages. In the 16th century Milan kept agents on Swiss territory to examine travelers on the St. Gotthard route.[3] This was a serious encroachment upon the sovereignty of a foreign power, but the fear of plague was such that it called for drastic measures. In the 17th century England required a bill of health of all ships sailing from Turkish and Egyptian ports.

Epidemiological intelligence was organized on a large scale during the 19th century when the Asiatic cholera invaded the Western world in repeated attacks. An international conference at which twelve nations participated met in Paris in 1851 for the purpose of securing international cooperation, particularly in the field of maritime quarantine. The conference failed to establish a permanent organization, but similar conferences were held thereafter, one of which met in 1881 at Washington where yellow fever was the chief topic of discussion. Finally, in 1909, the *Office International d'Hygiène Publique* was established in Paris with 54 nations participating. Epidemiological intelligence was its chief function, a function it shared from 1921 on with the Health Section of the Secretariat of the League of Nations.

Plague, cholera, yellow fever, and influenza are acute epidemic diseases which attack large groups suddenly and wipe out millions of human lives within a few years. Wherever they occur they present a strong challenge and, like war, they call for the mobilization of all the state power a society can muster. There are other less spectacular diseases; typhoid fever, dysentery, the many diseases that come from filth, contaminated water, bad food and general unsanitary conditions. These are a danger also, and equally in need of protective measures by the state power. The sanitation of man's environment was and still is an important function of government.

The administration of public health became an increasingly significant part of the general administration of the state. Laws and ordinances were enacted and enforced by the police and the courts. The physician was called upon in a dual capacity, as expert adviser to the legislator and as administrative officer. The protection of the people's health and the eradication of disease are tasks of such magnitude that they cannot be accomplished without the state power. Public health has been extending its field from century to century, and with the breaking down of barriers between preventive and curative medicine it is gradually developing into state medicine.

The administration of public health has always been influenced by two factors: the status of medical science and the prevailing political philosophy. The more that was known about the cause, nature and cure of disease, the more effectively a government could act. But the political philosophy determined whether a government was able to apply the existing knowledge, and in what way.

In the Western world two trends developed side by side from the 16th to the beginning of the 19th century. In countries with absolute government such as France, Prussia, Austria, Russia, the administration of public health was centralized and paternalistic, while much initiative was left to the local authorities in democratic countries where the prevailing philosophy was that of liberalism, such as England.

Under absolute government the monarch, advised by his cabinet, made the laws. He was to his subjects what in the family the father was to his children. In health matters he commanded what he considered good for the people and prohibited what he thought was bad for them. Enlightened despots, rulers like Frederick II of Prussia, Joseph II of Austria, or Catherine II of Russia surrounded themselves with the leading philosophers, scientists and physicians of the day. They listened to advice and the power they commanded enabled them to carry out far-reaching reforms. Of course, the people never had any guarantee that their monarch would be enlightened. Catherine II was succeeded by her half-crazy son Paul I; Joseph II by his brother Leopold II who pursued a reactionary course.

The chief exponent of this public health trend was Johann Peter Frank (1745–1821). Adviser to half a dozen monarchs, he was a physician and hygienist of great vision. In a six-volume work he studied the influence that the physical and social environment exerts on man's health, and he gave it the characteristic title *System einer Vollständigen Medicinischen Polizey*. He was a product of the philosophy of enlightenment, but he spent all his life in the service of absolute rulers. Fully convinced of the importance of social and economic conditions in determining the people's health,[4] his attitude nevertheless remained paternalistic: his ideal was a system of good health laws enforced by the police.

In England sovereignty lay with King, Lords, and Commons. Many acts of parliament were enacted on matters of public health. The liberal attitude—which in the course of the 19th century became dominant all over the Western world—had great advantages in that it encouraged individual initiative and open discussion, and protected the people against arbitrary power. Liberalism endeavored to promote health without excessive intrusion upon the individual's personal liberty. On the basis of this philosophy the great English public health movement was born towards the middle of the last century.

It is sometimes said that the German way in public health was to enforce health through the police while the English way consisted in acting through education and persuasion. There is some truth in the statement, yet it is a gross over-simplification of the facts. The English public health movement made full use of the state power. Around 1870 it was much easier to condemn dwelling houses as unfit for human habitation in England than it was in Germany. English local communities enjoyed a great deal of freedom, but the central government did not hesitate to bring pressure on them if conditions required it. Thus, about 1870 every community including a minimum of 300 taxpayers which in the preceding seven years had had an average death-rate of over 23 per thousand was forced to submit to a very strict investigation as soon as one-tenth of the taxpayers complained about health conditions. And according to the findings the communities were obliged to undertake certain measures.[5] Germany, on the other hand, could

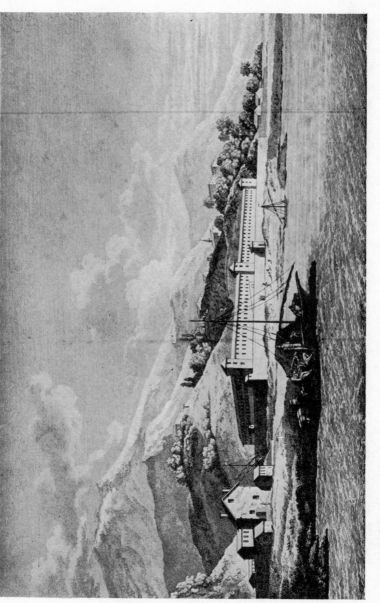

14. LAZARETTO IN GENOA. (From John Howard, *An Account of the Principal Lazarettos in Europe*, Warrington, 1789.)

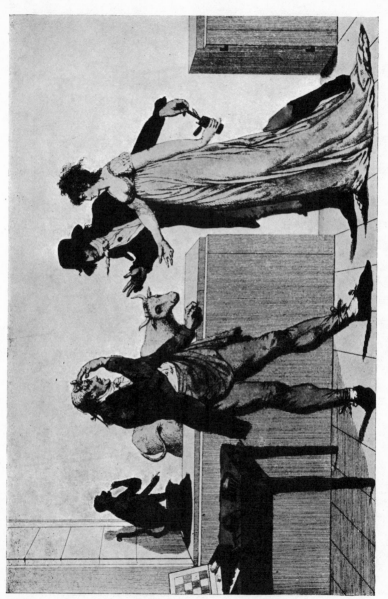

15. SATIRICAL PICTURE ON JENNER'S VACCINATION, 1801.

boast of some of the foremost pioneers of health education, men like Bernhard Christoph Faust (1755–1842) whose *Catechism of Health* was translated into English and published in Great Britain in five editions and in the United States in four editions.

The liberal attitude has serious limitations in the field of public health because it presupposes a standard of political education and a sense of social responsibility that few people possess. Quackery flourished in England more than in any other country. In Germany until 1869 medicine could be practised legally only by licensed physicians, but in that year the new *Gewerbeordnung*, the code regulating trades, permitted everyone who chose to do so, to give medical care and to collect fees for it, as long as he did not call himself a physician. Only licensed physicians were allowed to use that designation. This queer and at the time much criticized regulation was largely due to the liberalism of Rudolf Virchow, who justified it by declaring that the individual should have the freedom to select his own healer. He added that since the people were reasonable they would be able to differentiate between a genuine physician and a quack.

The limitations of liberalism were also apparent in the resistance to the enactment of vaccination laws in Anglo-Saxon countries and in several Swiss cantons. The individual's personal liberty was thought to be seriously endangered by forcing him to become sick artificially, if only slightly and for a few days, in order to protect him and others from really serious illness later on. The benefits, however, are so obvious and the discomfort suffered so small that a socially advanced population will unhesitatingly accept vaccination and other immunization techniques.

A misinterpreted liberalism is also responsible for resistance to the compulsory treatment of venereal diseases. The result is that their incidence is very much higher in such countries than it is in those where the treatment is free for everybody but obligatory.

Freedom is often confused with anarchy. In the highly specialized industrial society in which we live we all depend on each other, and we must learn to sacrifice minor liberties in order to preserve and safeguard the essential ones. Education is certainly most important in public health, for it teaches us not only how to live, but also how to pass and to obey laws that will protect the people's health.

The law has been called upon also to guarantee compensation for the loss of health.

Among primitive peoples and in all ancient civilizations a man who injured a fellow man was punishable. The most primitive reparation was provided by the *ius talionis*, "eye for eye, tooth for tooth, hand for hand, foot for foot." [6] Retaliation satisfied the desire for vengeance. It did not replace the lost organ nor did it compensate materially for it, but in the Code of Hammurabi as well as in the Laws of Moses it was the only admissible sanction among social equals. If, however, the victim was socially inferior, compensation in money took place. Thus the Code of Hammurabi prescribes: [7]

196. If a man has destroyed the eye of a Freeman, his own eye shall be destroyed.

197. If he has broken the bone of a Freeman, his bone shall be broken.

198. If he has destroyed the eye of a plebeian, or broken a bone of a plebeian, he shall pay one mina of silver.

199. If he has destroyed the eye of a man's slave, or broken a bone of a man's slave, he shall pay half his value.

200. If a man has knocked out the teeth of a man of the same rank, his own teeth shall be knocked out.

201. If he has knocked out the teeth of a plebeian, he shall pay one-third of a mina of silver.

In the Laws of Moses the man who injures his slave must compensate by letting him go free: [8]

And if a man smite the eye of his servant, or the eye of his maid, that it perish; he shall let him go free for his eye's sake.

And if he smite out his manservant's tooth, or his maidservant's tooth; he shall let him go free for his tooth's sake.

Compensation in money gradually became the rule also among social equals, but the amount to be paid varied according to social rank. Thus in the Hittite Code the breaking of a freeman's hand or foot cost 20 shekels of silver, but only half that amount if the victim was a slave. The penalty for breaking a freeman's nose was 1 mina of silver, and 3 shekels for that of a slave.[9]

In the case of murder or manslaughter the sanction was originally death: but even here compensation was accepted at a very early date and a slave, of course, could be replaced by another slave. According to the Hittite Code a man who killed a slave unintentionally had to replace him by giving another slave in his stead, but in the case of murder he had to give two slaves. For murder of a freeman the penalty was four slaves and two for manslaughter. The same Code already mentions compensation in money as being customary in certain regions.[10] The paying of *wergeld* instead of retaliation is found in many mediaeval codes.

In certain primitive tribes the man who killed a member of another tribe was not put to death but had to join the tribe of the victim. The murderer thus replaced the victim in person.[11]

Many ancient codes contain compensation tariffs. We find them in the Twelve Tables of Ancient Rome as well as in the *Lex Salica* and the Anglo-Saxon laws. They are interesting because they show the relative value attributed to the various parts of the body. Thus in the Code of Hammurabi the penalty for a broken bone or destroyed eye was 1 mina of silver, for knocked out teeth ⅓ of a mina.[12] In the Hittite Code the compensation for cutting off an ear was 12 shekels, for breaking a hand or foot, 20 shekels, but 1 mina or 60 shekels for cutting off a nose.[13] The fine was probably so much higher in the latter case because the injury seriously disfigured the victim.

The Anglo-Saxon laws have very elaborate tariffs. As an example

I wish to quote from King Æthelbert's Dooms, from which I have arranged injuries according to the amount of compensation to be paid: [14]

1 shilling: bruise, nail off, back molar

3 shillings: rib broken, exposure of bone, first molar, thumb nail off, smallest disfigurement of face, ear pierced

4 shillings: injury of bone, middle finger struck off, eye-tooth

6 shillings: arm broken, collar bone broken, ring finger struck off, front tooth, stabbing through arm, ear mutilated, nose pierced, greater disfigurement of face

8 shillings: forefinger off

9 shillings: nose pierced

10 shillings: great toe cut off

11 shillings: little finger struck off

12 shillings: thigh broken, belly wounded, ear struck off, speech injured, mouth or eye injured

20 shillings: chin-bone broken, thumb struck off, belly pierced through

25 shillings: one ear struck off, other hears not

30 shillings: shoulder lamed

50 shillings: foot cut off, eye struck out

The principle that an individual who had suffered an injury could bring suit for damage against the guilty person and thus recover for the tort was generally accepted throughout the centuries. It had its foundation in Roman law as well as in common law. The question became increasingly acute in the 19th century with the development of industry. As we discussed in a previous chapter, the new mode of industrial production made work infinitely more hazardous than in the past. Industrial accidents and occupational diseases increased considerably, and the question arose whether and under what conditions an injured workman could claim compensation from his employer.

The history of legislation on employers' liability and workmen's compensation is very interesting in that it reflects the political and social history of the period. In the beginning, legislation was all in favor of the employer, and the workman had hardly any chance of recovering for the damage done to him. Conditions changed when labor organized and became itself a political power. Under the pressure of organized labor, legislation was gradually liberalized so as to protect the worker's interests and promote his welfare, although this trend is still far from complete.

Under the common law a workman could obtain damages only if he could prove in court that the injury was due to negligence or fault of the employer.[15] It is obvious that it was extremely difficult for a workman to establish such proof as long as he was not protected by labor organizations. And if he succeeded in obtaining damages, most of the money was absorbed by the attorney's fee. The situation was made much worse by the so-called "fellow servant doctrine" which was first formulated in England in 1837 and was followed in the United States. According to this doctrine all individuals employed by a common master were considered fellow servants, and the employer was not held responsible for injuries resulting from the negligence or fault of any one of them. He was further exonerated if he could prove that the injured workman had been only partly negligent in the pursuit of his work. The law was, moreover, interpreted in such a way that the workman engaging in a hazardous occupation was assuming all risks ordinarily involved when he entered into a wage contract with the employer. Most vicious of all was a rule, in force in England until 1846 and in the United States even later, according to which the dependents of a workman who had suffered the worst, namely, a fatal accident, had no claim against the employer. The interpretation was that when the victim had died, the case had died also.

Conditions were somewhat better in those European countries that had codes based on concepts of Roman law. Thus the French *code civil* did not follow the fellow servant doctrine. The employer was liable for injuries due to his or his agent's negligence and had to pay damages for fatal accidents. However, in those countries also the worker had no claim for injuries due to ordinary risks or to his own negligence. In the middle of the century, at a time when both industry and its hazards were growing, the worker had very little protection against accidents and none at all against occupational diseases.

The development of the railroads created a new situation. The railroads were a dangerous means of transportation. Accidents were frequent, and as early as 1838, when the first line between Berlin and Potsdam was opened, Prussia made the railroad companies liable for accidents. Injured persons, employees and passengers, had to be compensated unless it could be proven that the injury was due to their own negligence or to an "act of God." Other states followed the example and after the unification of Germany an imperial statute enacted in 1871 extended the same liability to other industrial undertakings. This forced employers to seek protection by taking out insurance.

The English Employer's Liability Act of 1880 was a first step towards the abolition of the fellow servant doctrine. It had strong repercussions in the United States where the railroads had also been instrumental in changing conditions.

All the old liability laws had the serious shortcoming that they did not protect the workman against injuries due to ordinary risks or to their own negligence, and that they granted him damages only if he sued in court, a procedure that he usually could not afford. Gradually, and under pressure from labor, it was recognized that all industries, no matter how careful employer and employee might be, presented health hazards, that negligence of workmen was often nothing but the result of fatigue, and that it was not in the interest of society to have a legion of crippled workers dependent on charity. The view gradually crystallized that the compensation of workmen for injuries, irrespective of anybody's guilt or negligence should be considered part of the cost of production.

Once this view became prevalent, the time was ripe for a new type of legislation.

With Bismarck's social legislation Germany did the pioneering work in the field. The Sickness Insurance Act in 1883 guaranteed injured and sick wage earners medical treatments and cash benefits for 13 weeks of disability. The Industrial Accidents Insurance Act of 1884 established a system of compulsory insurance from whose funds employees were compensated for all injuries resulting from occupational hazards. In the beginning it applied only to industry and mining, but it was gradually extended to construction, transportation and agriculture. Enjoyed at first only by workmen, in 1929 compulsory insurance was extended to include office employees, and from 1925 on the system compensated not only for accidents but also for occupational diseases. The premiums were paid by employers only so that the cost was actually part of the cost of production. Advantages included treatment, rehabilitation, cash benefits in compensation for temporary or permanent disability, and pensions to widows.

The German Accident Insurance was a new departure, and the example it set was soon followed by a number of European countries. England's Workmen's Compensation Act of 1897 followed a somewhat different principle: it merely extended the employer's liability, forcing him to compensate injuries, but leaving insurance to his discretion. It did not provide compensation for injuries caused by "gross carelessness of the worker," so that law suits were unavoidable in many cases. When England revised its Compensation Act in 1906 thirty-one industrial diseases were included.

The United States was very late in enacting compensation laws. These followed the British pattern. By 1911 nine states had passed such measures; others followed in rapid succession, but there are still states that do not compensate for occupational diseases, and many of the laws now in effect have serious shortcomings.

Many people do not realize how hazardous industrial work is and what a heavy toll of life it still takes every year. According to the official report of the U. S. Department of Labor for 1939,[16] 18,000 workers were killed in that year, 106,000 sustained permanently disabling injuries and 1,407,000 sustained temporary total disability. Mining alone was responsible for 1,800 deaths. Agriculture, the least protected industry, had a death toll of 4,300 and 13,000 permanently disabling injuries. These figures show how necessary legislation is to prevent the victims of labor from becoming completely pauperized.

The law was also called upon to protect society against the physician. It would seem a paradox that society should have had to protect itself against the very men whose function it was to aid society, yet we must remember that the legal definition of the physician as one who is licensed by the state to practise medicine is relatively young, going back no further than the Middle Ages. Before that time anybody could call himself a physician, treat sick people accordingly and charge a fee for his services. Society was always aware that the physician's profession gave him a great deal of power over people. He knew drugs that could be used as remedies but also as poisons; he also knew secrets of his patients, and this increased his hold over them. Society tolerated the physician and his power because it had need of him, but at all times it endeavored to protect itself against misuse of this power.

The physician of primitive society, the shaman, was frequently under suspicion. It seemed logical that he who was able to remove spells should also be able to cast them. When no other culprit could be found, suspicion was often directed against the shaman, who had to submit to the ordeal or other means of divination if he did not choose to seek refuge in flight.

Most dangerous to society was an unskilled surgeon. The damage he could do was immediate and apparent to all. The first legal regulations we encounter were therefore directed against surgeons. The Code of Hammurabi made the surgeon liable for his actions; he was rewarded for successful operations but punished for unsuccessful ones. If, in operating on a slave he killed him, he was bound to replace him by another slave, and if as a result of an operation he destroyed a slave's eye, he had to pay half the slave's value in silver. If, however, a free man died as the result of an operation, the surgeon's right hand was cut off.[17] This stopped him once and for all. The law was so draconic that I doubt whether it was ever applied. No surgeon would ever have operated on a patient with such a threat hanging over his head or rather, his hand.

In ancient Persia we find prescriptions for the examination and licensure of surgeons. No surgeon was allowed to practise on Persians, on worshipers of Mazda, before he had performed three successful operations on infidels, on worshipers of the Daevas. If the three test operations had been unsuccessful he was declared "unfit to practise the art of healing forever and ever." And if he practised in spite of this prohibition and somebody died under his knife, he was punished for "willful murder." [18]

Neither the Greeks nor the Romans had any legal form of licensure. The public was not protected from charlatans, and there were plenty of them in Rome. A first step toward licensure was taken in the 2nd century A. D. when the considerable privileges extended to physicians in the Roman empire were restricted to a limited number of doctors which varied according to the size of the communities. Physicians had to apply for the privileges and present their credentials; thus the public knew that the privileged physicians, the *valde docti* or *archiatri* as they were later called, were real doctors who had satisfied the authorities as to their knowledge and skill.

The institution of our modern medical licensure which gives a legal definition of the physician is a creation of the Middle Ages.

It goes back to the Norman king Roger who in 1140 issued an order stating:

> Who, from now on, wishes to practice medicine, has to present himself before our officials and examiners, in order to pass their judgment. Should he be bold enough to disregard this, he will be punished by imprisonment and confiscation of his entire property. In this way we are taking care that our subjects are not endangered by the inexperience of the physicians.
>
> Nobody dare practice medicine unless he has been found fit by the convention of the Salernitan masters.

The old Norman codes were revived and extended by the Hohenstaufen emperor Frederick II who in his *Constitutiones Imperiales* issued from 1231 to 1240 regulated the practice of medicine in great detail. He prescribed a course of instruction of eight years: three years of logic and five of medicine, supplemented by a practical year. Candidates were examined by the most competent physicians, the Salernitan masters, in the presence of representatives of the state. After successful examination the *medendi licentia* was granted by the emperor or his representatives.[19] Thus the state assumed responsibility for the practice of medicine and guarded the people against the dangers resulting from the ignorance and incompetence of their doctors. A pattern was set which in the West was followed more or less closely to our own day.[20]

Society is legally protected from misuse of the physician's power in many other ways.[21] The patient who consults a physician enters into a contract that entitles him to sue the doctor for damage resulting from negligence. This is why physicians carry malpractice insurance. The doctor, on the other hand, as partner of the contract, can sue the patient for the payment of fees. The law protects the patient's secrets, a regulation that can be traced back to the Hippocratic Oath. Medical aid is in many cases impossible unless the patient has full confidence in his doctor and allows him to look into the secret places of the heart. There is, however, in the legislation of many countries a strong tendency to permit or even compel the physician to divulge secrets if the interest of society is involved.

The law protects germinating life and forbids abortion unless the pregnancy is a direct threat to the mother's survival. This is a Christian heritage. In antiquity abortions were performed frequently and in spite of the attitude reflected in the Hippocratic Oath; they were even recommended by such philosophers as Plato as a means of regulating the population. Christianity forbade abortion even if there was a medical indication for it, requiring that the physician sacrifice the baptized mother rather than the unbaptized infant, a view that the Catholic Church still holds, while the secular law fortunately has taken a different attitude.

The problem of abortion is serious. In pre-Hitler Germany it was estimated that the country annually lost more women from septic abortion than from tuberculosis. Wherever there is misery, where contraceptives are not easily available and a stigma is attached to illegitimate birth, clandestine abortions will always be performed. This is why the Soviet experiment in legalizing abortion was watched with great interest. As a matter of fact it was not an experiment but an emergency measure.[22] In 1920 conditions were very bad in Russia. Civil war and foreign intervention were still present; famine was ravaging parts of the country; women were taking an active part on the labor front and in the war; housing was poor, wages low, and contraceptives unavailable. Under these circumstances frequent abortions would occur which would greatly harm the women's health; it, therefore, seemed preferable to have the unavoidable abortions performed by competent physicians in hospitals.

Sixteen years later, in 1936, conditions had changed radically. Living and working conditions had greatly improved. The food shortage had been overcome completely, and wages were much higher. Already every second child was born in a maternity home, and there were enough nurseries available to take care of ten and a half million children. Birth control had developed and women could obtain information easily in the Women's Consultation Bureaus. Therefore, there was no longer any need for abortions, which are never quite harmless, particularly when they are performed repeatedly. The law was repealed, and at the same time large funds were appropriated for the construction of many additional maternity homes and nurseries, and for financial aid to large families.

What we can learn from the Soviet experiment is this: abortion is not needed and—unless there is some medical indication for it —can safely be forbidden as harmful to health in any society that (1) guarantees a job to all its members, men and women; (2) provides medical and social institutions for the care of mother and children free of charge; (3) gives adequate financial aid to large families; (4) provides contraceptive advice to all who seek it; and (5) attaches no stigma to illegitimate birth. When a society is unable to realize such conditions it must reckon with a large amount of clandestine abortions and many casualties. In such a case the legalization of abortion may be the lesser evil.

Another medico-legal problem that is still highly controversial is that of sterilization for eugenic reasons.[23] The development of medical and social services resulted in the preservation of hundreds of thousands of dysgenic individuals who in former centuries would have succumbed in the struggle for life. At the same time millions of the physically best equipped young men are killed off periodically in wars. This amounts to a negative selection and must ultimately result in a deterioration of the race.

Eugenics was a direct outcome of Darwinian theories. The idea of preventing unfit individuals from having offspring found a practical application as early as 1886 when August Forel, the Swiss psychiatrist, sterilized a woman who was suffering from a sexual neurosis. In 1892 he castrated individuals for purely eugenic reasons. Castration, however, was a serious matter because the operation upsets the endocrine balance. The new methods of sterilization inaugurated in 1897 and 1898 by Kehrer in Heidelberg and Ochsner in Chicago, namely, the severing, tying, or occlusion of the Fallopian tubes in the woman, of the *vas deferens* in the man, represented a great advance because they are relatively minor operations which have no ill after-effects.

As soon as sterilization began to be practised by physicians as a measure of preventing hereditary diseases, the legal question arose. Sterilization, obviously, could be abused. If society was to be protected, some legal regulation was necessary. The Catholic Church has always taken a very drastic stand against all forms of sterilization, finding its strongest sanction in the papal bull *Casti connubii* of 1930. Legislation, therefore, was enacted primarily in Protestant countries and, in Europe, first in the Swiss canton of Vaud in 1921. An amendment to the Public Health Act declared that an individual suffering from an incurable mental disease or from feeble-mindedness could be sterilized. The operation had to be authorized by the Public Health Council, which in turn would act after having sought the expert advice of two physicians.

In the United States Indiana enacted a sterilization law as early as 1907. It was declared unconstitutional in 1921, but new laws were passed in 1927 and 1931. The situation was similar in other states, and the question came before the Supreme Court in 1926. Chief Justice Oliver Wendell Holmes' opinion was very important. He said: [24]

> It is better for all the world if instead of waiting to execute degenerate offspring for crime or to let them starve for their imbecility, society can prevent those who are manifestly unfit from continuing their kind. The principle that sustains compulsory vaccination is broad enough to cover cutting the Fallopian tubes.

On the basis of this judgment the sterilization law of Virginia was declared constitutional and today 28 states have such laws.

Before 1933 a number of countries had the legal power to prevent manifestly unfit individuals from procreating offspring, but sterilization was applied on a very small scale. In the United States by January 1, 1937, only 25,403 persons had been sterilized, most of them in California. The situation changed when the Nazis came into power in Germany. Sterilization laws had been before the German Reichstag in 1907 and 1925, and the legislation that was finally enacted by the Nazi government in 1933 was based on thirty years of psychiatric and genetic research. The preparatory work was completed before Hitler came into power,[25] so that the law would probably have been passed sooner or later anyway. The Nazis, however, adapted it to their racial ideology, which was itself the frankly admitted basis of their health and population program. The Scandinavian countries enacted similar legislation,[26] but while they applied it slowly and cautiously, Germany went ahead immediately and on a tremendous scale. The law applied to individuals suffering from hereditary feeble-mindedness, schizophrenia, manic-depressive psychosis, epilepsy, and Huntington's chorea, from hereditary deafness and blindness, and from several genetically transmitted bodily malformations. The decision was in the hands of special so-called Hereditary Health Courts. In the first years of the regime over one quarter of a million individuals were sterilized, and it has been estimated possibly more on political grounds than on impregnable scientific evidence that the number of persons coming under the law would exceed 600,000.

It is too early to ask for convincing results, but I think it would be a great mistake to identify eugenic sterilization solely with the Nazi ideology and to dismiss the problem simply because we dislike the present German regime and its methods. The pioneering steps were, after all, taken by the United States and Switzerland,

and the Scandinavian laws are just as stringent as the German. The problem is serious and acute, and we shall be forced to pay attention to it sooner or later.

Another medico-legal question, the discussion of which comes up periodically, is that of *euthanasia,* the question whether the physician should be permitted to abbreviate a patient's final agony. It is a very delicate problem, hard to define in legal terms and, I think, is one of those problems that are better left to the individual conscience of the physician. It is very probable that euthanasia is actually practised by conscientious physicians much more often than we know.

There is one last relationship between disease and the law that I would like to discuss briefly. When a man steals somebody else's property or kills another individual, he is arrested, tried and jailed, or possibly executed. Society endeavors to protect itself against asocial individuals who break generally accepted rules, and until recently the sentence was intended to be a punishment. Society was taking vengeance, making the criminal suffer in retaliation for the offense he had committed. Gradually it was found that in many cases society was responsible for the asocial behavior of individuals whom it had deprived of educational opportunities, and of the chance to develop and apply their natural aptitudes. Adverse social and economic conditions, beyond the control of the individual, had distorted his sense of values and brought him into conflict with the law. The sentence passed by a progressive judge is framed with a view to re-educate and rehabilitate an asocial individual and to make him a useful member of society, but in the minds of conservative judges—and these, alas, are in the great majority—the primitive idea of vengeance and punishment is still very much alive.

Now, medicine has found that many individuals steal or kill or commit other crimes without being aware of what they are doing.

Their minds are disturbed as a result of illness and they are unable to distinguish between right and wrong at the moment they commit an offense. It must have been observed very early that in the course of fever diseases an individual became delirious, and that in his delirium he became violent and committed actions which he did not remember when the fever had receded. The same observation was made with persons intoxicated by alcohol or hashish or other drugs: our word *assassin* comes from the Arabic *hash-shash*, which means hashish eater.

The legal question arose whether such individuals could be held responsible for their actions and could be punished for deeds of which they had no knowledge. The law was always made for average people, for sane people able to distinguish between right and wrong. It was decided very early that people who are not sane are outside of society and therefore outside of the law. From the legal point of view, humanity was divided into two groups, the sane and the insane, those of the one responsible for their actions, those of the other not. Insane criminals were not punished, but since they were a menace to society they were formerly confined to jails, later to mental hospitals. The court, therefore, before taking further action, had in many cases to decide first whether an individual was sane or insane.

The question was of great importance, not only in criminal but also in civil law. A will written by a person who was not in full control of his mental faculties obviously could not be considered valid; insanity was a reason for divorce, for deposition of a monarch, for putting an individual under tutelage. In the Middle Ages already the courts called upon the physician to decide whether an individual was sane or insane, and the physician's expert testimony determined the action of the judges.

So far so good, but the trouble was that medical science was at all times at least half a century ahead of the law. This is perfectly normal because the law does not lead but follows. A medical discovery must first be accepted by the medical profession; then it must win general acceptance by society, and finally it may be embodied in a country's law. Legal reform is thus a very slow process. Now it happened that psychology and psychiatry developed a great deal during the 19th and 20th centuries. Pinel, who at the time of the French Revolution inaugurated a new era in psychiatry, was greatly interested in its legal aspects. In 1817 he published a treatise entitled *Résultats d'observations pour servir de base aux rapports juridiques dans les cas d'aliénation mentale*. His disciple Esquirol went even further and became a staunch defender of criminals who were mentally ill. In developing his theory of monomania he showed how individuals steal, kill, commit arson and sexual offenses as a result of irresistible impulses. In 1835 an Englishman J. C. Prichard introduced the concept *moral insanity*,[27] and in 1876 the Italian Cesare Lombroso published his famous book *L'uomo delinquente,* in which he discussed the fact that many criminals were mentally sick people. Freud and psychoanalysis finally unveiled a great many psychological mechanisms that threw further light on the asocial actions of individuals.

From the time of Pinel on, the law was increasingly bewildered by and resentful towards physicians, whom it frequently accused of endeavoring to prevent criminals from meeting with justly deserved punishment. For practical purposes the law, as we have seen, recognized only two categories, sanity or insanity, and required the physician to declare simply whether a man belonged to one or the other. The physician, however, knows that there is no sharp borderline between the two conditions and matters have gone so far that "insanity" today is a legal concept for which there is no precise medical equivalent. The psychiatrist who is called to testify in court, if he is an expert, gives his testimony in accordance with present psychiatric knowledge, while the court thinks and acts in terms of two generations ago. As a result, people who are obviously sick are sentenced to death and executed without knowing what is happening to them. On the other hand, mental patients who in the opinion of psychiatrists are a serious menace to society are often not confined to hospitals because their condition does not meet the legal definition of insanity. They are allowed to go free until they actually commit a crime.[28]

Conditions are unsatisfactory today and will probably remain so for a long time. One thing is certain, however, namely that experts called to testify should be real experts, not only physicians, but also trained psychiatrists with experience in legal matters. They should, in addition, be neutral, and to ensure this they should be appointed by the court and not by one of the parties involved.[29]

NOTES

1. Leviticus 15, 2 ff.
2. Numbers 5, 2.
3. Arnold Treichler, *Die staatliche Pestprophylaxe im alten Zürich*, Zurich, 1926, p. 40 ff.
4. See e. g. his oration "The People's Misery: Mother of Diseases," translated from the Latin, with an Introduction by Henry E. Sigerist, *Bulletin of the History of Medicine*, 1941, Vol. 9, pp. 81–100.
5. Max von Pettenkofer, *The Value of Health to a City*, Two Lectures Delivered in 1873. Translated from the German, with an Introduction by Henry E. Sigerist. Baltimore, The Johns Hopkins Press, 1941, p. 51.
6. Exodus 21, 24.
7. *The Hammurabi Code and the Sinaitic Legislation*, by Chilperic Edwards, London, 1921, p. 38.
8. Exodus 21, 26–27.
9. See Heinrich Zimmern, *Hethitische Gesetze aus dem Staatsarchiv von Boghazköi*, Leipzig, 1922, p. 7.
10. *Ibid.*, p. 5.
11. See A. S. Diamond, *Primitive Law*, London, 1935 and E. Sidney Hartland, *Primitive Law*, London, 1924.
12. *L.c.* § 198 and § 201, p. 38.
13. *L.c.* § 15, § 11, § 13, p. 7.

14. Albert Kocourek and John H. Wigmore, *Sources of Ancient and Primitive Law,* Evolution of Law, Vol. 1, Boston, 1915, pp. 516–517.

15. For this and the following see Edward Berman, Employers' Liability, in *Encyclopædia of the Social Sciences,* Vol. V, New York, 1931.

16. U. S. Department of Labor, Bulletin 625.

17. C. Edwards, *The Hammurabi Code,* London, 1921, §§ 215–223, pp. 39–40.

18. The Zend Avesta, I. The Vendidad, ed. by J. Darmesteter, in: *The Sacred Books of the East,* ed. by F. M. Müller, Oxford, 1880, vol. IV, pp. 83–84.

19. See Huilland-Bréholles, *Historia diplomatica Friderici Secundi,* vol. 4, Paris, 1854: Constitutiones Regni Siciliae. English translation in E. F. Hartung, Medical Regulations of Frederick the Second of Hohenstaufen, *Medical Life,* 1934, vol. 41, pp. 587–601.

20. See H. E. Sigerist, The History of Medical Licensure, *Journal of the American Medical Association,* 1935, vol. 104, pp. 1057–1060.

21. See L. Ebermayer, Der Arzt in Gesetz und Rechtsprechung, in: Der Arzt und der Staat, *Vorträge des Instituts für Geschichte der Medizin an der Universität Leipzig,* vol. 2, Leipzig, 1929, pp. 45–59.

22. See H. E. Sigerist, *Socialized Medicine in the Soviet Union,* New York, W. W. Norton and Co., 1937, pp. 246–253.

23. See S. Zurukzoglu, *Verhütung erbkranken Nachwuchses,* Basel, 1938.

24. Quoted from *Journal of Heredity,* 1927, vol. 18, p. 495.

25. Marie E. Kopp, Eugenic Sterilization Laws in Europe, *American Journal of Obstetrics and Gynecology,* 1937, Vol. 34, p. 499.

26. Denmark in 1929, Sweden and Norway in 1934, Finland in 1935.

27. A treatise on insanity and other disorders affecting the mind, London, 1835.

28. See Frederic Wertham, *Dark Legend; a Study in Murder,* New York, Duell, Sloan and Pearce, 1941.

29. See Winfred Overholser, Psychiatry and the Courts. Some Attitudes and their Reasons. *Virginia Medical Monthly,* 1940, Vol. 67, pp. 593–599.

CHAPTER V

Disease and History

WHATEVER we do becomes history the moment we have done it. In this chapter, however, we shall use the term in a much narrower sense and shall examine the influence of disease on some historical events.

Disease befalls individuals, and since individuals are the actors in the drama of history it may well happen that the illness of a man in a position of power influences his actions and thus has historical consequences. The same disease may also attack a large number of people at the same time, as happens when an epidemic invades the land. The results of such collective diseases that affect the life of entire groups are even more apparent. We shall, therefore, begin with the discussion of the historical consequences of some epidemic diseases.

There can be no doubt that few epidemics have upset the life of the Western world more deeply than the *plague*.[1] It is a disease of rats and other rodents caused by a bacillus that was discovered by Kitasato and Yersin in 1894. The bacillus can be transmitted to man by insects such as fleas, and once it has taken hold among human beings it spreads by contact from man to man following the highways of traffic. Chronicles often report that plague broke out after some great natural catastrophe, a drought, flood or famine. Such reports are not due to the desire for dramatizing events but have a sound rational foundation. When granaries are empty and basements are flooded, the rats move closer to men, and if there happens to be an epidemic among the rodents the chances of human contamination are great.

The plague occurs in two forms, bubonic and pneumonic. In the first case the lymphatic glands, particularly of the groin, armpit and throat, swell and present what was commonly called the *plague bubo*. Abscesses develop; pus is discharged which is highly virulent. Patients recover or die from septicaemia, from general blood poisoning. In the case of pneumonic plague the bacilli invade the respiratory organs; pneumonia develops and frequently kills people within a few days. The dead are livid, hence the name *black death*. The season often determines the type: bubonic plague being more frequent in summer, pneumonic plague in winter.

It is striking that the historical period that we call the Middle Ages begins and ends with the only two great pandemics of plague that Europe has experienced. The beginning of the Middle Ages is usually set with the beginning of the migration of nations in the 4th century. The invasion of the Roman Empire by barbarian tribes was undoubtedly a far-reaching event. They destroyed a great deal, but they also preserved much. Roman civilization was still strong enough to subjugate the invaders. In the beginning of the 6th century the Ostrogoths ruled Italy, but Theodoric's administration was essentially Roman. The offices at his court were Roman offices held by Romans. There still was a Roman senate and there still were Roman consuls. Roman *civilitas* was Theodoric's ideal. Cassiodorus, the last great Roman scholar, lived at his court, and there died Boëthius, the last Roman philosopher and scientist.

And then the plague invaded Italy. It came from the Orient, was in Constantinople in 532 at the time when Justinian I was on the throne, whence it is usually called the plague of Justinian. Spreading west, it arrived in Italy and soon was all over Europe. Many places were attacked several times, and it seems that the epidemic was complicated by a violent outbreak of smallpox. According to contemporary chronicles the devastation was terrific. There are, of course, no statistics but it may well be that in the course of a few decades a large section of the European population was wiped out.

After the plague Italy presented a totally different picture. The empire of the Ostrogoths was destroyed. The Lombards were in power. Their administration was Germanic and so was their law. The Pontifical State had taken shape and was becoming a political power. Gregory the Great was made pope in 590. Benedictine abbeys were spreading over the Western world.

Similar transformations took place in the East. Justinian considered himself a Roman emperor, and he actually was the last Roman emperor, the goal of whose policy was no less than the restoration of the Roman Empire in all its former grandeur. He thought of himself as the natural superior of all the barbarian kings who were ruling on Roman territory. He wished to combine military glory with legislative deeds and had the Digest of Roman Law compiled. Like the Roman emperors of old, he embellished his capital with gigantic buildings such as the Church of St. Sophia. After the plague the Eastern Roman Empire had collapsed; the successors of Justinian were no longer Romans but Byzantines, and Greek had replaced Latin as the language of the administration.

And if we look further east we find that great transformations were in the offing there also. In 571 Mohammed was born in Mecca.

Thus the 6th century marks a turning point in the history of the Mediterranean world, and the great plague of Justinian appears as a demarcation line between two periods. An old civilization was coming to an end: still alive in all its external features, it had lost its creative power—why, we do not know and can only speculate. The plague in its repeated waves killed millions of people, caused untold suffering. The administrative machinery, vacillating as it was, collapsed under the onslaught in many places. Ambitious political plans were frustrated. The old world broke down, and on its ruins a new civilization began slowly to rise.

The mediaeval world experienced no further pandemics of plague for many centuries. This is astonishing because there were frequent outbreaks in the near East and the traffic between East and West was very lively, particularly at the time of the Crusades. There were sporadic cases, a few local epidemics, but they never spread although there were plenty of rats in the mediaeval town and sanitary conditions were by no means good. And then, in the 14th century, in 1348, the plague again made one of its world-shaking onslaughts. This time it was called the Black Death.

From 1315 to 1317 Europe experienced one of its most devastating famines. In the city of Ypres which at that time numbered 20,000 inhabitants, 2,794 corpses were buried in the summer of 1316.[2] Europe had hardly recovered when the plague made its invasion of the continent. Again it came from Asia and moved westward in three large thrusts directed against the Black Sea, against Asia Minor and Greece and against Egypt and North Africa. It attacked southern Europe, moved north along the western coast, turned east, encircled central Europe, and then broke in upon it from all sides. When a city was stricken, the disease usually resided in it for a period of four or six months, killed off a large section of the population and disorganized the entire life of the town.

Estimates of the casualties vary from 25 to 40 millions. It is very likely that Europe lost between a quarter and a third of its entire population. Florence lost 60,000 inhabitants, Strasbourg 16,000, Basle 14,000, Padua two-thirds, Venice three-quarters. Two hundred thousand villages and farmholds were entirely depopulated.

The effects of a catastrophe of such magnitude were obviously far-reaching. Psychologically people reacted by either throwing themselves into licentiousness and dissipation, or more often by making penance and resorting to asceticism. The sect of the Flagellants was revived, particularly in Germany, and enjoyed a vogue until Pope Clemens VI stopped it. The Jews were persecuted, particularly in southern Germany, and were burned in their houses by the thousands. Whenever there is a great calamity, people seek a scapegoat. Noblemen and municipalities were heavily indebted to the Jews, and the plague gave them an opportunity to get rid of their despised creditors.

When the plague broke out, wars were raging all over Europe, but the disease very effectively interrupted them, at least for a while. France and England were engaged in the war that was to last almost a century and leave both countries thoroughly exhausted. England, equipped with the new firearms, had defeated the French at Crécy and had conquered Calais after a siege of eleven months. The plague forced them to withdraw and compelled them to sign a truce. The Scottish allies of France who intended to invade the north of England were not only defeated by the English troops but also decimated by the plague. The Kingdom of Naples was saved by the plague which forced the Hungarian army of occupation to a hurried retreat. In Spain, in Germany, in Poland and Russia, in the Byzantine empire, everywhere military operations were interrupted or entirely stopped by the epidemic.

The most far-reaching effects were probably felt in the economic life of the continent. As a result of the many casualties, a very serious shortage of labor developed and the consequence was a long period of high prices. This is why England passed the Statute of Labourers in 1350 and France in the following year issued a royal ordinance on the subject. The intention of both was to lower prices by regulating wages.[3] Civil unrest followed in many countries; peasant revolts occurred in France and England, while in Flanders the crafts rose against the patrician regime of the cities.

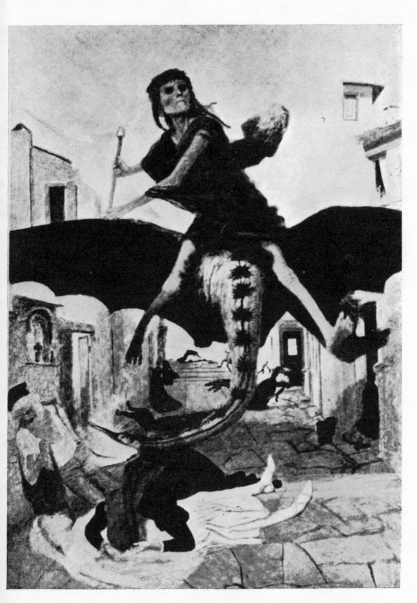

16. THE PLAGUE. (Painting by Arnold Böcklin. Basle Museum.)

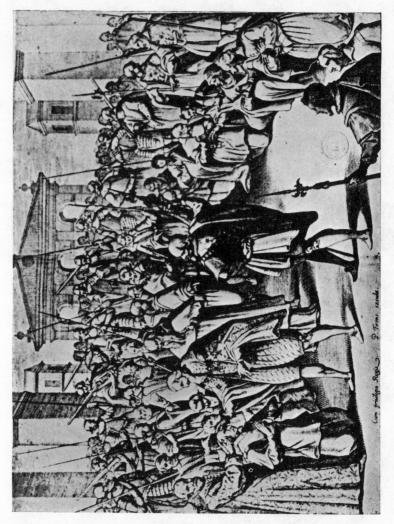

17. THE KING'S EVIL. Henry IV of France touching scrofulous patients. (Engrav-

Mediaeval economy had been steadily expanding until the 14th century, when it became static and began to show signs of disintegration. As Pirenne pointed out very justly, the great catastrophes that befell the century, famines, pestilence, wars and social unrest, were largely responsible for such a development. Thus the Black Death, the century's greatest disaster, played an important part in clearing the way for the rise of a new economic order which was to become the foundation of a new period in European history.

When the plague invaded Europe, Petrarch was in Avignon, a city that suffered a great deal from the epidemic. Pathetically he exclaimed: "Has one ever seen anything like this, ever heard reports of a similar occurrence? In what annals has one ever read that the houses were empty, the cities deserted, the farms untended, the fields full of corpses, and that everywhere a horrible loneliness prevailed." [4]

Boccaccio was in Florence at the time of the Black Death and in the introduction to his *Decameron* he gave a very graphic account of it, writing, not in Latin, but in the vernacular, in Italian. In other words, the men who stood at the threshold of the Italian Renaissance were contemporaries of the plague which in the 14th century as in the 6th occurred at a turning point of European history.

Hans Zinsser in his very witty book *Rats, Lice and History* [5] has a chapter entitled "On the Influence of Epidemic Diseases on Political and Military History, and on the Relative Unimportance of Generals." The point is well stressed because history shows over and over again that the best prepared campaigns broke down under the impact of epidemics and the lack of medical services. The establishment of well organized army medical corps is a relatively recent development, and generals were only too inclined to regard the army surgeon as a necessary evil and a nuisance, as a man who was always ready to interfere with their plans. It has been recognized only very recently that medical science is one of the most important elements of strategy.

From the Renaissance on, *typhus* was one of the most dangerous enemies ever to defeat brilliant armies and play havoc with the civilian population of many countries. Typhus is caused by a small micro-organism, the *Rickettsia,* which lives in lice and is transmitted by them. Hence the disease becomes a menace whenever sanitary conditions are bad and people are exposed to the louse. In war filth accumulates and it is difficult for the soldiers to keep clean. Typhus was also a great problem in times of economic depression and in the crowded and unsanitary prisons of the past. Hence the disease was also called camp fever, jail fever or hunger typhus.

In the Renaissance it was considered a new disease although it was probably not new to Europe. Typhus came originally from the East, and cases must have occurred in Europe in the Middle Ages although the disease was not recognized as an entity of its own.[6] There is no doubt that an epidemic broke out in the Spanish army of Ferdinand and Isabella during the siege of Granada in 1489 to 1490. It was then described as a "malignant spotted fever," and the assumption was that the disease had been brought by soldiers who had come from Cyprus where it was considered very common.

Typhus also played the decisive part in the second war between Charles V and Francis I of 1527–1529. The pope, Clemens VII, was allied with France. The Imperial army of Charles V marched triumphantly through Italy, sacked Rome and made the pope a prisoner. The tide turned when the plague broke out in Rome and decimated the invaders. At the same time the French army was pushing through Italy. Finally the Imperial troops were besieged in Naples. They were starved out and their cause seemed lost when suddenly typhus broke out among the besieging troops and the

118

French army was almost wiped out. In 1530 in Bologna the pope crowned Charles V ruler of the German Empire, and Zinsser is justified in saying that this last coronation of a German emperor by a pope occurred "by the power of Typhus Fever." [7]

The disease was from now on and for a long time to come the steady and dread companion of armies. It could no longer escape the attention of the physicians. Girolamo Fracastoro, the most distinguished epidemiological writer of the period, gave in 1546 a classical description of it in his *De contagione et contagiosis morbis eorumque curatione libri III*. According to him the disease had first occurred in Italy in 1505 and 1528 but was known to be common in Cyprus and other islands of the Eastern Mediterranean. What struck the people most was that patients suffering from this fever had red spots on their chest, back and arms. Hence they called the disease *lenticulae* or *puncticula* because the spots looked like small lentils or flea bites. Before Fracastoro another Italian physician, Geronimo Cardano, had already spoken of flea bite fever, but this was in a book that had not the authority of that of Fracastoro. [8]

From the Renaissance to our days typhus has played a great part in the shaping of historical events. In 1552 it was not an ally but a foe of Charles V when it forced him to abandon the siege of Metz. In the first part of the Thirty Years' War, from 1618 to 1630, typhus was the major catastrophe. What soldiers did not destroy, the disease did. In the second part of the war plague was in the foreground, and of course dysentery, typhoid and scurvy were never missing. [9] It took Central Europe a century to recover from the blows of famine, war and pestilence.

The louse was still triumphant in the 18th century, and in almost every European war of the period, including the campaigns of Napoleon, more people died from typhus than from battle wounds. Conditions changed in the second half of the century. In the battle between soap and the louse, the latter for the first time was forced to retreat. Typhus disappeared from most western European countries, and armies could destroy each other without interference. Typhus, however, remained endemic in Ireland and in eastern Europe, that is in countries with a lower standard of living. In Mexico and the southern part of the United States the disease had prevailed for centuries and still occurs in a milder form. Whether it existed in America before the Spanish conquest or whether it was imported from Europe is still controversial, but there are good arguments for the theory of a pre-Columbian typhus.

At the time when the World War of 1914–1918 broke out, medical science had made such tremendous progress that it was hoped that the war could be fought without major epidemics. This was actually the case on the Western front, but on the Eastern front typhus required only three months to make its appearance and to establish itself as the chief strategist of that sector. It broke out in Serbia in November 1914 and reached its climax in April of the following year. A mortality that was 20 per cent. in the beginning reached 60 and even 70 per cent. at the height of the epidemic.[10] Typhus killed Serbs and Austrian prisoners, soldiers and civilians alike; it devastated Serbia and for a long time prevented the Central Powers from occupying the country. Throughout the war typhus prevailed on the Eastern front but was kept within bounds owing to the energetic delousing of troops—until it swept Russia in an unprecedented epidemic from 1918 to 1922.

Typhus was an enemy well known to the Russians. In the twenty years before the Revolution the country had an average of 82,447 registered cases annually. Whenever there was a famine or a crop failure, the morbidity more than doubled. During the war the disease spread slowly but steadily; in 1915, 154,800 cases were registered, but the great epidemic broke out toward the end of 1918 and invaded the country from three centers: Petrograd, the Roumanian front and the Volga region. As a result of civil war and foreign intervention health services had broken down in many sections of the country. A famine assailed the Volga region and set the population in motion. The epidemic reached its climax in 1920, declined in 1921, and flared up again in 1922, chiefly in the famine districts. It is difficult to give accurate figures because the registration of diseases obviously breaks down when a country is torn by civil war, but it is safe to estimate that in the four years from 1918 to 1922 between twenty and thirty million cases occurred and that ten per cent. succumbed.[11] For a while it looked as if the fate of the Revolution was at the mercy of typhus and in 1919 Lenin said: "Either socialism will defeat the louse, or the louse will defeat socialism." It was an uneven fight because as a result of foreign boycott there was a serious shortage of the two most necessary commodities, soap for cleanliness and fuel for disinfection. A tremendous effort was made nevertheless. The railroad lines were watched and quarantine stations were established at all junctions; passengers were taken from trains, were bathed and disinfected, and sick persons were isolated. "Bath weeks" were organized during which entire sections of a town were cleaned and disinfected.

At the same time other epidemic diseases were raging: relapsing fever, cholera, dysentery, and malaria spread from the Caucasus to the Arctic zone. It was a picture such as the world had not seen since the Middle Ages; and if plague had broken out in addition to the other diseases, it is very likely that entire sections of Russia would have been completely depopulated.

Now that the Second World War is being fought and is involving territories where typhus is endemic, the spectre of a major epidemic is constantly threatening. At the moment these lines are being written, in the spring of 1942, reports of localized and minor outbreaks have been received; but it seems that the disease is still under control, and it is very probable that it will remain so for some time. Medical services have been greatly improved in all armies. The Red Army is equipped with special bath-trains consisting of nine cars with all facilities for bathing, washing and disinfection, and they are sent right into the front lines.

The actual danger will come later when the war enters its next phase, when the liquidation of Fascism will lead to revolution and open civil war. Then typhus may again raise its head and play its traditional rôle in the shaping of history.

Let us look at another disease different in character from those discussed so far, but one which has also had a deep influence on the life of nations, *malaria*.

In 1880 Laveran discovered in Algeria the protozoa that cause the disease by invading the blood stream. Soon thereafter they were also described and further investigated in Italy by Marchiafava and Celli. In 1895 Ronald Ross found that the parasites are transmitted to man through the bite of Anopheline mosquitoes. These classic discoveries explained a great deal. They explained the relation between the intermittent fevers and swamps, the breeding grounds of mosquitoes, and showed why the vicinity of marshes had always been considered unhealthy places for human habitation. They also explained the seasonal character of these fevers which would always flare up in the summer and autumn. Stimulated by these discoveries, some extremely interesting historical studies were made, of which I would like to discuss only two.

In 1909 W. H. S. Jones, one of the foremost students of Greek medicine, published a very challenging book, *Malaria and Greek History*.[12] His thesis was that the Greeks who surrendered to the Roman legions were not the same who had fought off the Persian invaders and that the changes which had taken place were primarily due to malaria. He describes these changes in the following words: [13]

Gradually the Greeks lost their brilliance, which had been as the bright freshness of healthy youth. This is painfully obvious in their literature, if not in other forms of art. Their initiative vanished; they ceased to create and began to comment. Patriotism, with rare exceptions, became an empty name, for few had the high spirit and energy to translate into action man's duty to the state. Vacillation, indecision, fitful outbursts of unhealthy activity followed by cowardly depression, selfish cruelty and criminal weakness are characteristic of the public life of Greece from the struggle with Macedonia to the final conquest by the arms of Rome. No one can fail to be struck by the marked difference between the period from Marathon to the Peloponnesian War and the period from Alexander to Mummius. Philosophy also suffered, and became deeply pessimistic even in the hands of its best and noblest exponents. "Absence of feeling," "absence of care,"—such were the highest goals of human endeavour.

Jones, of course, does not deny that other factors may have played a part, such as admixture of foreign population, the growth of idleness, luxury and vice, and the loss of a vigorous religious faith; but he thinks that a strong healthy people reacts against such factors and overcomes them. Malaria, however, saps the vitality of the people and destroys their very stamina, as can be seen today all over the world.

It is very difficult to determine the prevalence of a disease when statistics are non-existent and the literature preserved is fragmentary. Jones, by examining carefully the ancient non-medical and medical writers, came to the conclusion that there is only the slightest evidence that malaria existed on the mainland of Greece in early times; that the disease was probably common around 500 B. C. in Magna Graecia and on the coast of Asia Minor; and that it invaded the mainland in the second half of the 5th century, thus probably leading to a serious outbreak in Attica during the Peloponnesian War. And finally, around 400 B. C. malaria would have been endemic throughout the greater part of the Greek world.

The effects of malaria on the population were again, in Jones' own words, the following: [14]

(1) The rich, the capable and the energetic seek healthier homes, and so the inhabitants of a malarious district tend to become a mere residue of the poor and wretched.

(2) Cities being, as a rule, less malarious than cultivated plains, the urban population tends to absorb the agricultural class, and national physique and well-being suffer in consequence. Cities isolated by malarious surroundings often fall into decay and ruin.

(3) This process will be accompanied by great economic loss, for extremely fertile districts, which are the peculiar prey of malaria, may fall altogether out of cultivation. The ruin of agriculture is a great blow to any country, and it must be remembered that malaria attacks farmers in particular, and that mostly at harvest-time, when all their energies are specially needed.

(4) Malaria falls most heavily upon the young, whose physical powers are so weakened by repeated attacks of fever that childhood may be one long sickness, and adequate education impossible. *Aestate pueri si valent satis discunt.* The inhabitants of malarious districts age rapidly and die young.

(5) Exertion and strain often bring about a relapse, because the malaria parasite will live in the body for months, or even years. Naturally, the inhabitants of malarious places tend to avoid fatigue, and to become sluggish and unenterprising. A habit of laziness is gradually formed.

(6) Account must also be taken of the loss of life, loss of time and the physical suffering caused by the disease, besides the permanent psychical disturbances it may produce in the patient.

Jones' thesis is extremely interesting. There can be no doubt that the prevalence of malaria must have adversely affected the Greeks, as it does every population even today when we possess specific remedies in quinine and its substitutes. Until the 17th century there was no cure and the disease was permitted to take its natural

124

course. Whether the effects were as far-reaching as Jones assumes is questionable, but malaria certainly was an important factor in the later history of Greece.

It was important also in determining the history of another region, the Roman Campagna, the land that surrounds the city of Rome. Angelo Celli, one of the great malaria epidemiologists, who spent all his life combating the disease in Italy, made an extensive study of the history of the Campagna.[15] He was struck by the fact that this region was at times a complete desert and at other times a flourishing landscape, teeming with life. He found that in the course of twenty-five centuries the Campagna was inhabited and flourishing in four periods (1) in the pre-Roman era; (2) when Imperial Rome was at the height of its power; (3) in the early Middle Ages [8th and 9th centuries]; and (4) in modern times from the 15th to the 17th centuries. Between these periods the Campagna was a place of desolation, with ruined and abandoned hamlets and a few wild sheep grazing under the walls of the eternal city. Emperors and popes made great efforts to repopulate the region, offering premiums and subsidies to settlers, but it was all in vain. What is the explanation?

It was often assumed that the many wars that afflicted the city of Rome were responsible for the devastation of the Campagna, a very inadequate explanation because once a war is over life returns rapidly to the very battlefields, particularly in the environs of a great city. Celli undoubtedly hit the right answer when he made malaria responsible for the vicissitudes of the Campagna. It was malaria which at times made life impossible, killed or weakened the people and drove them from the land; it was malaria, in another parasitic form, that killed horses and cattle and laid the land bare. Celli's historical studies showed that in certain regions malaria occurs in periodic cycles. The disease takes hold of a region, develops, and drives all life away. *Dea febris* reigns supreme. And then after centuries, for reasons not yet known, the disease gradually recedes and life returns. There is no doubt that malaria was the history-making factor in the Roman Campagna.

The great part played by this disease in the colonization of America has recently been demonstrated in a most illuminating study.[16]

From these few examples it has become evident that collective diseases, chronic or acute, endemic or epidemic, have played an important part in the history of mankind. But other diseases have also had their impact on history, and I would like to mention in this connection the queer relation between *scrofula* and the institution of royalty.

Ancient gods performed miracle cures by touching patients. Asclepius appeared to sick people sleeping in his temples, and the touch of his hands healed them. Herophilus called medicinal drugs "hands of the gods." The Roman emperors had divine character, were worshiped like gods, and of some of them we hear that they performed cures. In the ancient Orient the monarchs were anointed, and the holy oil gave them divine power. The rite was continued in Judaism and was taken over in the Middle Ages. The Merovingian Pepin the Short was the first French Monarch to be anointed: this made him king by the grace of God and gave him divine power. The same rite was adopted in England toward the end of the 8th century and was soon generally applied all over Western Europe.

Once the king was anointed, he became the "Christ of the Lord." A crime against His Majesty was a sacrilege. Through anointment he shared in the divine power and when he touched a sick man, God healed him. Miracle cures are related of many of the early kings in France as well as in England, but the curing of scrofula by the royal touch seems to have been initiated in France by Philip I (1060–1108), in England probably by Henry I (1100–

1135).[17] Why scrofula and no other disease became the *mal du roi* or the *King's Evil* is not known. At any rate this faculty of the kings of France and England to cure scrofula became a carefully guarded attribute of royalty. When Charles I of England was kept in prison, numerous patients wanted to be touched by him and the House of Commons appointed a committee to prepare "a Declaration to be set forth to the People, Concerning the Superstition of being Touched for the Healing of the King's Evil." Royalists later even claimed that Cromwell had usurped the privilege of touching scrofulous people. When Charles was beheaded, handkerchiefs were dipped into his blood and some people believed that these relics still had the power of healing.

The rite was continued in England with interruptions until the reign of Queen Anne. On April 27, 1714, three months before her death, she performed the ceremony for the last time. Thereafter it was never repeated in England but was continued in France and even survived the Revolution. At the time of the Restoration, in order to give royalty its mediaeval prestige, Charles X was persuaded to perform the traditional rite. He did so once, in 1825, but this was the end of it.

The kings of England, and they alone, had another magic healing power. On Good Friday they made offerings of gold and silver at the altar under the Cross, purchased them back and had rings made from them. These *cramp-rings,* as they were called, had the faculty to cure people suffering from all kinds of cramps and particularly from epilepsy. The rite was established in the 14th century and followed the vicissitudes of its predecessors.

When a man in a position of power suffers from a disease, his actions may be affected by it. A toothache is extremely irritating, a headache or a cold is oppressing; pneumonia prostrates a man, and this may happen at a crucial moment when he is expected to

127

make far-reaching decisions. The question is therefore justified whether physical ailments have not had more influence on historical events than we commonly expect.

Tolstoi in his great novel *War and Peace* raises the problem and discusses it in great detail.[18] Many historians had claimed that the battle of Borodino on September 7, 1812, was not won by the French because Napoleon was suffering from a cold. Had he not had a cold, his disposition during the battle would have been much more ingenious, Russia would have been destroyed *et la face du monde eut été changée*. If such a view were correct, Tolstoi argues ironically, then the butler who on September 5 forgot to give Napoleon his watertight boots, would have to be considered the savior of Russia. Tolstoi also refers to a remark that Voltaire once jokingly made, namely, that the Massacre of St. Bartholomew's Day had taken place because Charles IX had had an upset stomach. He very justly opposes and ridicules such naive conceptions. His own view on causality in history is that the course of world events is predestined by a higher power, by the concurrence of all individual wills having a share in these events, so that Napoleon's part at Borodino was merely on the surface. In order to stress his point he gives a very fine analysis of the psychological situation in which the French army found itself at that moment.

History is made by individual human beings, to be sure, and whether they are healthy or sick, sane or insane, makes a difference. Yet the place an individual holds, the power with which he is invested, and the use he is permitted to make of his power, are determined by a great variety of factors, by social and economic conditions first of all, but also by hopes and fears, ambitions and frustrations and other psychological factors. There are potential men of genius, potential heroes and villains in every country at all times. Conditions determine whether they remain in the dark or come to the fore, to what purpose and on what scale they apply their activities. Disease of an individual and even a deadly disease

128

does not alter the course of history. A cause may collapse *when* the leader dies, but not *because* of his death. It collapses only when the forces that carried the leader have lost their momentum. Otherwise, his death may even activate the cause, as history has demonstrated more than once.

NOTES

1. The literature on the history of the plague is very extensive. The following are some of the basic books that should be consulted in this connection. Georg Sticker, *Abhandlungen aus der Seuchengeschichte und Seuchenlehre*, I. Band: Die Pest. Erster Teil: Die Geschichte der Pest. Giessen, 1908.—F. A. Gasquet, *The Great Pestilence (A.D. 1348-9), Now Commonly Known as the Black Death*, London, 1893.—Anna Montgomery Campbell, *The Black Death and Men of Learning*, New York, 1931.—Albert Colnat, *Les Épidémies et l'Histoire*, Paris, 1937.—See also Henry E. Sigerist, Kultur und Krankheit, *Kyklos*, Jahrbuch des Instituts für Geschichte der Medizin an der Universität Leipzig, 1928, vol. 1, pp. 60–63.

2. See Henri Pirenne, *Economic and Social History of Medieval Europe*, New York, n.d. [1937], p. 195.

3. *Ibid.*, p. 195 f.

4. *Epistulae de rebus familiaribus*, VIII, 7.

5. Boston, 1935.

6. The early testimonies have been collected by Heinrich Haeser, *Lehrbuch der Geschichte der Medicin und der epidemischen Krankheiten*, vol. III, Jena, 1882, pp. 357 ff.

7. *L.c.*, p. 253.

8. *De malo recentiorum medicorum medendi usu libellus*, Venice, 1536. It was later incorporated in his *De Methodo Medendi Sectiones Tres*. The passage appears as Caput XXXVI of Sectio Prima.

9. Gottfried Lammert, *Geschichte der Seuchen, Hungers- und Kriegsnoth zur Zeit des Dreissigjährigen Krieges*, Wiesbaden, 1890.

10. See Zinsser, *l.c.*, p. 297.

11. See L. Tarassevitch, Epidemics in Russia since 1914. Report to the Health Committee of the League of Nations. Epidemiological Intelligence, No. 2, March 1922 and No. 5, October 1922.

12. Manchester University Press, 1909.

13. *L.c.*, p. 102.

14. *L.c.*, pp. 107–108.

15. Angelo Celli, *Storia della Malaria nell'Agro Romano*, Memorie della R. Accademia Nazionale dei Lincei, Città di Castello, 1925. An abbreviated English translation was published under the title *The History of Malaria in the Roman Campagna from Ancient Times,* London, 1933.

16. St. Julien Ravenel Childs, *Malaria and Colonization in the Carolina Low Country 1526–1696*, Baltimore, 1940.

17. The best critical study on the subject is Marc Bloch, *Les Rois Thaumaturges,* Publications de la Faculté des Lettres de l'Université de Strasbourg, Fascicule 19, 1924.

18. Vol. IV, Part X, Chapter 28.

CHAPTER VI

Disease and Religion

WHAT is disease? Why does a man suddenly act and react differently from other people, feel handicapped in the performance of his physiological functions, and suffer? To us disease is a biological process. It takes place in the human body and may be localized in a certain organ, but since all organs are inter-related and form an organic whole, it is always the whole organism that is affected. And since body and mind are one, disease is experienced not only physically but also mentally.

The concept of disease as a biological process is relatively young, and disease can be and has been interpreted in very different ways. Primitive man found himself in a magical world, surrounded by a hostile nature whose every manifestation was invested with mysterious forces. In order to live unharmed, he had to use constant vigilance and had to observe a complicated system of rules and rites that protected him from the evil forces which emanated from nature and his fellow men. Magic was the means that gave him power over his surroundings, and everyone had to acquire some skill in magic if he wanted to live in harmony with the world, to make it a well integrated part of his physical and social environment.

When a man became sick, there was a reason for it: somewhere, somehow his vigilance had broken down and a stronger power was in command. A fellow man had bewitched him, or a spirit had taken possession of his body. The primitive concept of disease was magical. It contained religious elements, to be sure, but at that stage of civilization it is difficult to draw a line between religion and magic. Primitive medicine also knew of many procedures that we consider rational such as massage, sweat baths, or bloodletting, and the drug lore of many tribes was quite extensive. But these seemingly rational treatments were applied as part of a magical ritual: a drug did not act as a drug but because the ritual under which it was given, the incantation pronounced over it, gave it power to cure disease and alleviate suffering.

Thus magical, religious and empirical elements are inextricably blended in primitive medicine under the common denominator of magic. This gives it a character of its own, basically different from the medical systems of civilized societies. Likewise the primitive medicine-man cannot be compared with the modern physician. He is different and has many more functions: [1] he cures diseases but also makes rain; he is often the bard of the tribe and sometimes its chief; he is the man who has more knowledge than any other tribesman because he knows the traditions and has mastered magic, and he uses his knowledge to protect the tribe and make it prosperous.

With developing civilization the components of primitive medicine began to evolve along their own lines. They were still combined in Babylonian medicine, but the accent had shifted from magic to religion. Babylonian medicine was an elaborate system of religious medicine.[2] All disease came from the gods, and the task of the priest-physician was to discover and interpret the intentions of the gods so that he could placate them. Babylonian medicine included a great many magical and also empirical elements, but as a whole it was a system of religious medicine.

In ancient Egypt the three elements of primitive medicine are still found side by side, but the split has gone further. We have purely rational and purely magical medical texts. The Edwin Smith Papyrus,[3] a 16th century B. C. copy of a much older text, is en-

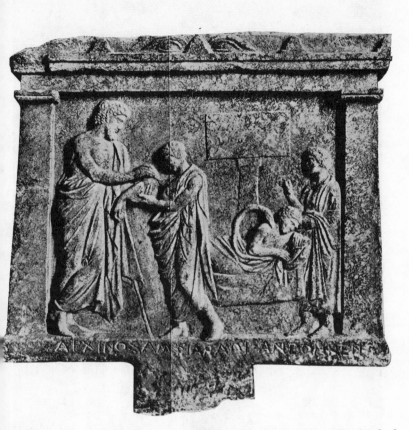

8. MIRACLE CURE IN A TEMPLE OF AMPHIARAUS. (Relief
rom Attica. National Museum, Athens.)

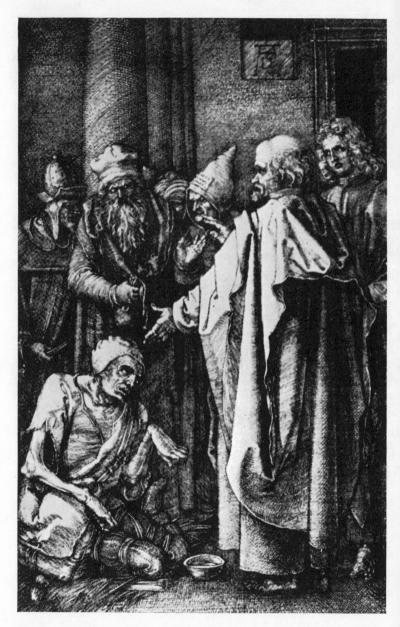

19. ST. PETER CURING THE LAME. (Engraving by Albrecht Dürer.)

tirely rational. The incantations at the end are undoubtedly inter-
polations. Its rational character may to a certain extent be due
to the fact that the Edwin Smith Papyrus deals primarily with
surgical affections. The Ebers Papyrus,[4] written in the 15th century B. C. is a purely medical book dealing with internal diseases.
It begins with a prayer to Isis, just as Arabic medical books begin
"In the Name of God the Merciful the Clement." There are incantations, but they are relatively rare, and as a whole this papyrus
also describes a rational system of medicine. Its chief content consists of an enumeration of diseases and disease symptoms, with
prescriptions for pharmacological treatment. In a significant passage the papyrus mentions three types of healers, namely, the
physician, the Sachmet-priest, and the exorcist.[5] We find the exorcist at work in some of the younger papyri, such as Papyrus
Brugsch Minor,[6] which is purely magical; it discusses diseases of
women and children and gives most elaborate magical prescriptions. We know from other literary and archaeological sources that
religion and magic played a very important part in Egyptian life.

The split between the elements of primitive medicine was complete from the Greek period on. The 6th century B. C. marks a
turning point not only in the history of Western thought but also
in the history of medicine. Rational systems of medicine developed
that consisted not merely of collections of crude empirical facts
—lists of symptoms and recipes—but endeavored to interpret the
nature of health and disease. They were based on observation and
experience, excluded mythology and the transcendental, and interpreted the problems of medicine philosophically, and later scientifically. How people ever succeeded in liberating themselves from
the bonds of magic and religion when they approached problems
of health and disease is still a mystery. The fact that they did suc-
ceed gives the Greek genius its unique position. The task was
easy for younger civilizations because they were able to follow a
pattern that was transmitted to them by the Greeks.

In spite of the development of rational medicine, religious and even magical medicine never died. All the elements of primitive medicine have survived the centuries and millennia to our very days. At all times the three systems could be found side by side, sometimes in peaceful competition, sometimes in open conflict. When the dominating philosophy was rational, science flourished and religious medicine was in the background, to satisfy the mystical desires of a minority and serve as a last refuge for patients for whom scientific medicine had failed. Magic in such periods was relegated to the uneducated and "unenlightened" elements of the population, living in peasant superstitions and in accepted customs and habits the original meaning of which had been forgotten. In many countries people still carefully observe lucky and unlucky signs without knowing that the interpretation of *omina* was once a highly developed science.

When a mystical philosophy prevails, as in times of great physical or social catastrophes, religious and magical medicine come to the fore. Fear obliterates reason. People revert to primitivism and endeavor to ward off by magical means the evils that are threatening them.

While Greek physicians and philosophers pondered over the nature of disease, there were many people who interpreted illness in religious terms and sought healing in temples. Evil was sent by the gods, and so was disease. The darts of Apollo brought pestilence, the snake-haired Furies punished crime and induced raving madness. The glance at Medusa paralyzed, and her picture was worn as an amulet to protect a person from the evil eye.

All ancient gods had the power of healing. Zeus was worshiped as Zeus Soter, and in Rhodes as Zeus Paian. Hera appears as Hera Sotira or Telexinia, in Rome as Juno Sospita. In Lemnos, the earth upon which Hephaestus fell became the *terra Lemnia sigillata* which was used as a remedy for snake bite and mania. Pallas

Athena was invoked in Athens as Athena Hygeia, in Kyzikos as Athena Iasonia. In Sparta, people suffering from eye diseases worshiped Athena Ophthalmitis. Apollo was considered the inventor of medicine: his healing functions were denoted by a great variety of attributes such as akesios, alexikakos, epikourios, iatros, iatromantis, paion, soter.

Thus whoever suffered from disease could go to almost any temple, bring offerings and pray for the restoration of his health. Gradually, however, religious medicine crystallized in the cult of Asclepius.[7] For centuries it was the foremost healing cult, spreading from Epidauros all over the Greek world and reaching Rome in 291 B. C. Originally the physicians' patron, Asclepius was gradually exalted and deified. Legends arose that made him the son of Apollo, the disciple of the centaur Chiron, and his temples became places of pilgrimage sought by the sick and afflicted.

Even in ruins Epidauros is still an imposing sight. Walking through the ruins with Pausanias as a guide, we can reconstruct the place as it was when many generations of patients, Greeks and Romans, visited it. The center of the holy place was the temple where stood the gold and ivory statue of the god. His bearded face had a mild and kind expression as he stood leaning on his staff, a helper to the afflicted. He was the only Greek god whose life had been pure and holy, the only god about whom no scandalous stories were told. Some day he was to become the chief competitor of Christ.

We still see the ruins of a large hostel built around four courtyards for the accommodation of the pilgrims. The theater, a gigantic structure, is one of the best preserved Greek theaters. A concert hall, a stadium, and baths were provided for the entertainment of the visitors. The holy shrine was fenced in, for only pure people were allowed to enter: for the impure, menstruating women, women in childbirth, and the dying, a Roman senator, Antoninus, had donated a special house outside the precincts.

The healing act was the so-called *incubatio*. This took place in the *abaton*, galleries located not far from the temple. Patients, after having undergone preparatory rites, went to sleep in these galleries. The god appeared to them in their dreams and when they woke up, they were cured—at least some of them, those of whom we have records. Failures are usually not advertised. A number of Epidaurian tablets relating such miraculous cures have been preserved from the 4th century B.C. They tell us of an Athenian woman, Ambrosia by name, who was blind in one eye. She could not believe that lame and blind people could be cured by mere dreaming. But then, when her night came, the god appeared to her. He promised to cure her but wanted her to donate a votive offering to the temple. It was to be a silver pig in memory of her stupidity. Whereupon the god cut open the eye, rubbed in balm, and when it was day she was cured. Or we read of Agestratus who was cured of headaches so severe that he was never able to sleep. Another patient, Gorgias, had a suppurating wound in the chest which had been made by an arrow: he woke up with a sound skin and holding the arrow point in his hand.

We know today the psychological mechanism of suggestion and are using it consciously. There is no doubt that suggestion and auto-suggestion can remove certain disease symptoms. Faith, the tension of religious fervor, create a state of mind that is most favorable to therapy. It has always been a special type of patient that sought healing in cults: chronic patients as a rule and many of them neurotics. The symptoms of hysteria respond most easily to such treatment, but the cure is not a permanent one: the basic disease condition remains unaffected. It is very probable that Ambrosia left the temple seeing with both eyes, but it is quite possible that a few months or a few years later she became deaf or lame, or showed some other hysteric symptom. And Agestratus, who lost his headaches at Epidauros, may well have developed pains in the stomach instead.

It cannot be denied, however, that organic diseases may also be cured by suggestion. Every cell, after all, is under the influence of the nervous system. I remember a very prominent dermatologist who suffered from a chronic eczema that drove him almost mad. He consulted the greatest authorities in the field, tried every conceivable treatment without any result. Finally in despair, he went to see Émile Coué, a layman in Nancy whose treatment by autosuggestion was then in great vogue—and he was cured. Being a scientist he sought a rational explanation for his own case. He found that suggestion had not cured the disease but had removed the atrocious itching. The eczema, left to itself without the constant irritation caused by scratching, healed spontaneously.

It is well known that warts, a contagious affection, react very easily to suggestion. Warts are therefore extremely popular in all kinds of healing cults. A case that occurred in the practice of one of my European classmates is a classical example. He is a pediatrician and was treating a girl who among other things had several ugly warts on her fingers. It was decided that they should be cauterized with nitric acid. When the day came, mother and child were sitting in the waiting room. The girl was very apprehensive and nervous, and a woman who happened to be waiting in the same room inquired what the trouble was. When she was told about the warts and the impending treatment, she warned the mother not to have nitric acid applied because it was painful and left scars. She knew of a better treatment. Her instructions were: "Buy a new silk ribbon. Make as many knots as the child has warts. Drop the ribbon in the vicinity of a school where many children pass by. A girl will pick up the ribbon and with it your daughter's warts." It was not very charitable advice, but it was effective. The child actually lost her warts.

The case is a good example of the survival of primitive procedures in 20th century folk medicine. The ribbon must be new and of silk. In other words it must cost some money and is a sacrifice. The disease is fastened in the ribbon through the magic knots. And finally a transplantation takes place from one individual to another.

Modern experience has shown that not only nervous but also certain organic diseases can be greatly improved if not cured by suggestion and other forms of psychotherapy, and we must bear this in mind when we study the "miracle cures" that took place at Epidauros and in other healing cults. Without such results religious medicine would have died out. Just as pleasant experiences are remembered for a long time while unpleasant ones are repressed, successful cures are carefully recorded while failures are soon forgotten.

In the 5th century B. C. while Hippocratic medicine flourished, the cult of Asclepius was established in Athens and soon thereafter in other Greek communities. There was no conflict between the two forms of medicine, which flourished side by side. In the centuries of imperial Rome the cult was widespread and very popular. A tide of mysticism swept over the ancient world. Miraculous cures were performed not only by Asclepius but also by Cybele, Dionysus, Osiris, Serapis, Mithras, and patients flocked to their temples. Chief competitor, however, was a new Syrian sect that had come with the promise of healing and redemption—Christianity.

At the time of Christ the healing of the sick played such an important part in all cults that the new religion could not have competed with them unless it had also held the promise of miraculous healing. The Gospels relate a great number of cures. They are the miracles most frequently performed by Christ. He healed demoniacs, the blind, lepers, paralytics, people suffering from various other chronic diseases or infirmities, and even resuscitated the dead. He cured by virtue of the divine power that was in him. An episode in Mark 5, 25–34 is enlightening in this respect. A woman who "had an issue of blood twelve years" and had been unsuccessfully treated by many physicians, touched Christ's garment: "And straightway the fountain of her blood was dried up; and she felt in her body that she was healed of that plague. And Jesus, immediately knowing in himself that virtue had gone out of him, turned him about in the press, and said, Who touched my clothes?" The same idea is expressed in Luke 6, 19: "And the whole multitude sought to touch him: for there went virtue out of him, and healed them." He cast out devils "by the Spirit of God." [8]

Sometimes a profession of faith was required of the sick. The two blind men who wanted to be cured by the son of David were asked: "Believe ye that I am able to do this? They said unto him, Yea, Lord. Then touched he their eyes, saying, According to your faith be it unto you. And their eyes were opened." [9] Another blind man he cured saying: "Receive thy sight: thy faith hath saved thee." [10]

Sometimes Christ cured people by touching them with his hands, the classical gesture of miraculous healing. He touched the eyes of the blind,[11] or he spat on them and put his hands upon him.[12] In another case he spat on the ground, made clay with the spittle and anointed the eyes of the blind man with the clay.[13] In very many cases the cure was effected by mere command, by the magic of the word. To the leper Christ said: "Be thou clean," [14] to the paralytic: "Rise, take up thy bed, and walk," [15] to the man whose hand was withered: "Stretch forth thine hand." [16]

Like the other miracles, the cures attributed to Jesus amazed the people. They made the works of God manifest [17] and proved that Jesus was the Messiah, the Christ. The Gospels set a pattern that determined the forms of religious medicine in the Christian world for many centuries. Not only Christ had the faculty of performing such cures but his apostles also. "Then he called his twelve disciples together, and gave them power and authority over all devils, and to cure diseases. And he sent them to preach the kingdom of God, and to heal the sick." [18] Peter cured a lame man by saying to him: "In the name of Jesus Christ of Nazareth rise up and walk." [19] Paul and the other apostles performed similar cures. They were considered the most forceful demonstration of the power of God and played an important part in the conversion of pagans. The ancient world fully believed in miracles. Asclepius and the other gods performed them, while the philosophers Plotinus and Apollonius of Tyana were said to have wrought miraculous deeds.[20] Just before Julius Caesar was murdered, all the doors and windows of his house opened up spontaneously, strange noises were heard, ghosts gleaming like red-hot metal were seen fighting each other.[21] Such stories circulated among the people and were believed by many: why should they not equally believe in the Christian miracles? All saints performed them. The *Legenda Aurea* is full of reports of miracle cures; they repeat each other in endless monotony.

Medicine was faith healing in the early Christian community. When a man was sick, the elders of the church prayed over him, "anointing him with oil in the name of the Lord. And the prayer of faith shall save the sick, and the Lord shall raise him up; and if he have committed sins, they shall be forgiven him." [22] Greek medicine was a pagan art for which there was no room in the early church. In the 2nd century A. D. Christian students of Galen were excommunicated. Gradually, however, a reconciliation took place. When Christianity became the official religion of the Roman state it had to compromise with necessity by taking over the cultural heritage of the past. Christians became physicians and treated patients by applying the doctrines of pagan medical writers. Medical books were copied in Benedictine monasteries; hospitals were erected for the stranger, the poor and the sick.

The rational medical systems of antiquity were saved. They survived the centuries, were assimilated and integrated into Christian theology. Galen became a dominating authority but for centuries little progress was made. In a world in which the church played an overpowering rôle and in which religion permeated all aspects of life, religious medicine was close to the people and was bound to be very much in the foreground. It assumed more definite forms which reflected many pagan elements.

When a man was sick he made offerings and prayed for healing, addressing himself, not to God directly, but to the Virgin Mary and to the saints, asking them for their intercession. On votive paintings Mary is frequently represented kneeling before God and showing her breasts to remind him that she had borne his son. She was worshiped in many forms: as *medicus infirmorum, medica humanarum infirmitatum, aegrorum curatio, medicina aegrotantibus, vulnerum nostrorum medicina, auxilium festinum in morbis, dolorum omnium finis, remedium nostrum, medicina nostra.*[23] In France alone about forty churches were dedicated to her in her healing capacities, Notre-Dame des Malades, Notre-Dame des Infirmes, Notre-Dame des Langueurs, Notre-Dame du Remède, Notre-Dame de Guérison, Notre-Dame de Convalescence, Notre-Dame de Santé, etc.[24] Most famous of all today is Notre-Dame de Lourdes where on February 11, 1858, the Virgin Mary appeared to Bernadette Soubirous, and four days later a miraculous spring appeared. Hundreds of thousands of patients make pilgrimages to Lourdes every year, and water from the sacred spring is shipped all over the globe. Lourdes is to the Catholic world what Epidauros was to the ancients.

Among the saints an interesting specialization took place. As we mentioned before, they all had performed miracles, and the early saints who had converted pagans and died as martyrs for their faith all had miracle cures to their credit. They all had the power to pray and intercede with God for a sick man. Gradually, however, saints became specialists whose help was invoked in the case of definite diseases. Thus, from the 7th century on, St. Sebastian became the patron saint who protected men from the plague. The Plague of Justinian in the 6th century that had caused so much misery and suffering had created a strong demand for a helper. Sebastian became a plague saint as a result of his legend. Diocletian had him shot by his archers, and according to the legend he was pierced by so many arrows that he looked like a hedgehog. And yet he was not dead. Darts, however, had always symbolized the sudden death from pestilence; Apollo sent the plague by shooting arrows at people. Sebastian, being stronger than the death caused by arrows, became the redeemer from the plague. This cult started in Pavia in 680 at the time of an outbreak of plague when his relics were brought from Rome and an altar was erected to him in the church of San Pietro in Vincoli.[25] In the 14th century the plague again ravaged the world and millions of people died in spite of St. Sebastian. This created a demand for a new plague saint who appeared in the form of St. Roch, a citizen of Montpellier who had devoted his life to the nursing of the plague-ridden. From then on, both saints were invoked in times of pestilence.

In a similar way St. Lazarus was the patron saint of the lepers, St. Vitus of those suffering from epilepsy and other spastic diseases; St. Anthony cured those suffering from ergotism, St. Blaise those afflicted with throat diseases. An endless list of saints could thus be drawn up.[26] Their help was greatest at the places where they were buried. Every one of their relics and even their images had miraculous power. Medals of them were worn as amulets. And when patients had been cured by their intercession, votive offerings representing the organ from which they had been suffering were often given to the church, just as had been done in pagan antiquity.

Throughout the Middle Ages and for long thereafter people ascribed epidemics to the wrath of God and endeavored to placate Him. Mental patients were considered possessed by the devil and were exorcised. The uterus was conjured lest it should wander through the body and cause hysteria.[27] Everywhere the ancient magical rituals were applied in Christianized form.

The Reformation discarded the pagan elements that had invaded the Christian church. It marked a return to the Gospel and to the simplicity of life of the early Christian community. The cult of the Virgin Mary and of the saints, the worship of relics and images, the pilgrimages to holy shrines—all these were abandoned. Thus the elaborate rituals of religious medicine were discarded, but there was a need for some kind of equivalent in Protestantism. This was discovered in the simple way of prayer as outlined in the Epistle of James. When a man was sick he prayed to God directly for healing, or fellow members of the community came and prayed with him. If he had faith he had hope. Healing was faith healing.

Religious medicine was systematized in various ways within Protestantism and several churches developed that emphasized the healing aspects. Most widespread among them was the so-called Christian Science, which was founded by Mary Baker Eddy (1821–1910). Her history is well known. Born in New Hampshire, she suffered from various ailments until she found her savior in Phineas Parkhurst Quimby who must be regarded as the spiritual father of the whole movement. He was a watchmaker in Maine who saw a Frenchman work some magnetic cures. The theory of animal magnetism elaborated by Franz Mesmer (1734–1815) was meant to be scientific, but actually was a wild speculation. Mesmer differentiated between mineral and animal magnetism. He assumed that an infinitely subtle substance permeated the entire cosmos, and that this substance was responsible for the influence exerted by bodies on each other, a phenomenon that he called animal magnetism. Disease was the result of disturbed magnetism and could be cured by magnetic means. In the therapeutic ritual that Mesmer developed, hypnosis and suggestion were the most important elements and the whole theory enjoyed a great vogue in the early 19th century.

Quimby undertook magnetic cures but soon discovered that the procedures usually observed were quite unnecessary, that faith was sufficient in itself. He cured Mary Baker, who then became his disciple; after his death in 1866 she carried on his work and from it developed her own doctrine. In 1875 she published her book *Science and Health with Key to the Scriptures*. She moved to Boston where the Mother Church was founded. The sect grew and has today over one thousand churches in the United States with close to a million adherents.

Christian Science is not a therapeutic system but a religion. Its strongest appeal to the people, however, probably rests in its promise of healing not only sickness but every sort of evil. For evil does not exist at all. There is no matter but only spirit. Spirit is God. God is good and omnipresent. Sickness, sin, death, do not exist. They are human errors. When a person is sick, he is in error. When he is brought back to correct thinking, he will necessarily feel well again.

Christian Science became popular at a time when American medicine was developing an extremely mechanistic approach to disease and was neglecting psychological factors. There was a gap into which Christian Science stepped. Conditions have changed today. Medical psychology and psychiatry have developed and are taking an increasingly important place in scientific medicine. As a result, the Christian Science movement has stopped growing. It will remain because it satisfies the mystical needs of a minority which is always found in a society like ours, until some other movement will take its place.

Christ sent his apostles "to preach the kingdom of God and to heal the sick." The Protestant Church still preaches the kingdom of God, but it left the healing of the sick to the physicians. It was felt sometimes that the Church was neglecting one of its tasks by leaving medicine entirely in the hands of the physicians. Christian Science deliberately took the patient away from the doctors. A movement of a totally different kind developed in the beginning of

144

our century with the Emmanuel Church. The founder, Elwood Worcester, a minister of the church, had studied psychology with Wundt in Leipzig. He was a friend of the Philadelphia neurologist S. Weir Mitchell and became greatly interested in the field of mental diseases. As Rector of the Emmanuel Church in Boston, he began around 1905 to hold a Tuberculosis Class in cooperation with Dr. Joseph H. Pratt, addressing himself to the sick slum-dwellers for whom there was no room in sanatoria. "The treatment consisted of the approved modern method of combatting consumption, *plus* discipline, friendship, encouragement and hope, in short a combination of physical and moral elements." [28] The example was widely followed and the next step was the establishment of the Emmanuel Health Class for work among "the nervously and morally diseased."

The movement was in no way antagonistic to scientific medicine. On the contrary, it cooperated with leading physicians and admitted patients only after they had been examined by a doctor. It was in other words psychotherapy, mostly suggestion, applied by the minister instead of the doctor and making use of religious elements. There is no doubt that many patients suffering from neuroses were cured or at least improved by such methods. One must not forget that in America in those days the average physician had little psychiatric experience and well-trained psychotherapists were not very numerous.

Today the American doctor is a physician of body and mind alike. His training includes psychology and psychiatry, and there are many specialists available. They appreciate the cooperation of the minister whenever a patient happens to be a religious individual. Faith undoubtedly is an important therapeutic factor, whether it be faith in science, in religion, or in both. It is safer, however, to have mental clinics operated by medicine than by the church.[29]

Scientific medicine has progressed a great deal since the days of Asclepius, but it still has serious limitations. There continue to be many phenomena of disease that science cannot explain and many diseases that it can neither prevent nor cure. Most people still die from disease rather than from the degenerative processes of old age. As long as medicine has not reached its goal of eradicating disease there will always be patients who, hoping for a miracle, will seek help in religion or even in magic. Whenever the physician underestimates the importance of social and psychological factors in the genesis of disease and in its treatment, he will find a competitor in the priest who appreciates these factors.

NOTES

1. See the excellent article of Erwin H. Ackerknecht, Problems of Primitive Medicine, *Bulletin of the History of Medicine,* 1942, Vol. XI, pp. 503–521.

2. Henry E. Sigerist, *Medicine and Human Welfare,* New Haven, 1941, p. 2 ff.

3. James Henry Breasted, *The Edwin Smith Surgical Papyrus,* 2 Vols., Chicago, 1930.

4. *The Papyrus Ebers, the Greatest Egyptian Medical Document,* translated by B. Ebbell, Copenhagen, 1937.

5. Papyrus Ebers 99, 2–3.

6. Adolf Erman, *Zaubersprüche für Mutter und Kind aus dem Papyrus 3027 des Berliner Museums,* Berlin, 1901.

7. An exhaustive study on Asclepius by Emma and Ludwig Edelstein is in course of publication at the Johns Hopkins Press.

8. Matthew 12, 28.

9. Matthew 9, 28–30.

10. Luke 18, 42.

11. Matthew 20, 34.

12. Mark 8, 22–26.

13. John 9, 6.

14. Matthew 8, 3.

15. John 5, 8.

16. Matthew 12, 13.

17. John 9, 3.

18. Luke 9, 1–2.

19. Acts, 3, 6.

20. R. Reitzenstein, *Hellenistische Wundererzählungen*, Leipzig, 1906.

21. Plutarch, Caesar.

22. James 5, 14–15.

23. See Alphonse-Marie Fournier, *Notices sur les Saints Médecins*, Solesmes, 1893, p. 17.

24. *Ibid.*, p. 18.

25. See Henry E. Sigerist, Sebastian-Apollo, *Archiv für Geschichte der Medizin*, 1927, vol. XIX, pp. 301–317.

26. See Dietrich Heinrich Kerler, *Die Patronate der Heiligen*, Ulm, 1905.—Adalberto Pazzini, *I Santi nella Storia della Medicina*, Roma, 1937.

27. Werner Bernfeld, Eine Beschwörung der Gebärmutter aus dem frühen Mittelalter, *Kyklos*, 1929, vol. 2, pp. 272–274.

28. Elwood Worcester, Samuel McComb, Isador H. Coriat, *Religion and Medicine, The Moral Control of Nervous Disorders*, New York, 1908, p. 1.

29. See in this connection Charles Reynolds Brown, *Faith and Health*, New York, 1924.

CHAPTER VII

Disease and Philosophy

THALES OF MILETOS, who flourished in the 6th century B. C., was the first Greek philosopher. He never wrote a book but was remembered for having declared that moisture was the primary cause of all things. This short statement marks the beginning of European philosophy. The naive observer contents himself with noticing the reality of things and perhaps endeavors to make practical use of them. Thales, however, reflected about things. Daily experience taught him that everything had a cause, and so he concluded that the world also must have a cause and he sought for an explanation of the world. His approach to nature was what the Greeks expressed with the verb *theorein*. He looked at things without taking them for granted but in ever renewed astonishment, and the explanation he gave was not mythological as previous interpretations had been. He had observed that all living beings are moist, that animal sperm is moist, that there are deserts where there is no water. On his peregrinations he had seen the effect of the inundation of the Nile. And he concluded that moisture must be the primary cause of things.

Other explanations were given. Anaximander declared the limitless and Anaximenes the air to be the primary element. They both wrote books *On Nature*, which they sought to investigate, and they both were also interested in practical problems. Anaximander was said to have constructed a globe of the heavens, to have drawn a

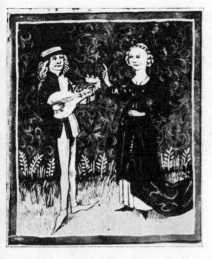

20. THE PHLEGMATIC.

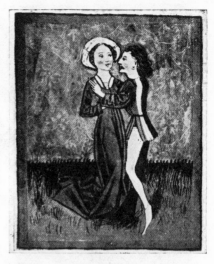

21. THE SANGUINE.

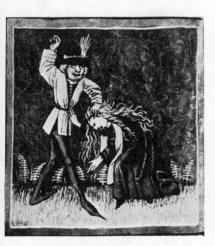

22. THE CHOLERIC.

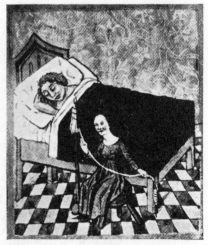

23. THE MELANCHOLIC.

THE FOUR TEMPERAMENTS. (From Zurich manuscript C54/719, 15th century.)

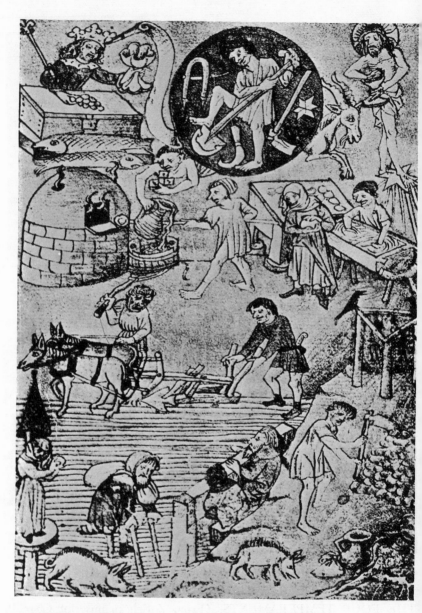

24. THE CHILDREN OF SATURN. (From Tübingen MS. M.d.2, early 15th century.)

map of the world, and to have introduced the sun-dial from Babylonia. Anaximenes engaged in astronomical studies.

Gradually these early investigators and philosophers of nature extended their studies to the problems of health and disease, and in this development the school of Pythagoras played a very important part. As a result of political conditions Pythagoras emigrated from Samos to southern Italy, and in Croton he was soon surrounded by disciples. The members of the school believed in the transmigration of souls and sought redemption from the cycle of incarnations by leading a pure life. They submitted to a strict mental and physical diet which was designed to make them resistant to all kinds of disturbances. If, however, a disorder had developed, they tried to restore the lost balance physically with medicine, mentally with music. Medicine and music were thus drawn into the circle of their investigations.

In the course of their studies the Pythagoreans observed that there was a definite relation between the length of a string and the note it gave off when it was plucked. They concluded that harmony was a mathematical proportion, and Number appeared as the essence of all things. The numbers in their systematized balance formed a symmetry, and the ideal number was 4, not 5 or 7. Two pairs of numbers with opposite qualities seemed to constitute a perfect harmony. Later Empedocles taught that the world was built of four elements, earth, water, air and fire. These combined and separated, attracted and repulsed by the basic forces of Love and Strife.

We begin to perceive in what direction medicine will move. In the 6th and 5th centuries schools of physicians had developed in the Greek colonies, in southern Italy, Sicily, and Asia Minor, particularly in Cos and Cnidos. They were not schools in our modern sense, with buildings, laboratories, clinics, and a charter, but rather free associations of physicians and their apprentices. Many of their writings are preserved in the collection that was later attributed to

Hippocrates. They all had to raise and try to answer the questions: What is health? What is disease?

The answers varied a great deal, but they all had something in common. They excluded magic and mythology. Disease is not the result of witchcraft, nor the work of evil spirits sent by the wrath of revengeful gods. It is a natural process, not basically different from the processes of normal life. Man in health and disease was part of nature, and had to be studied and interpreted like other natural phenomena with the methods that had been developed by the pre-Socratic philosophers.

Health appeared as a condition of perfect equilibrium. When we are in good health we breathe freely, digest our food, excrete urine, move and think as a matter of course, without being aware of it. But this equilibrium can be upset by atmospheric factors, faulty diet, wrong mode of living or other conditions. And this upset balance manifests itself in pains, fever, swellings, disturbed functions and other symptoms of disease.

Such an explanation, correct as it was, was yet too vague to be of much use in medicine, and physicians had to decide which were the essential constituents of the body that balanced each other in health. According to some it was the *dynameis,* the forces that are active in the organism. According to others it was the humors, blood, bile, urine, and the like. In one of the younger Hippocratic writings, *On the Nature of Man,* we find the beginnings of a theory that was to exert a tremendous influence on medicine for over two thousand years. We read that there are four cardinal humors in the human body: blood, phlegm, yellow bile, and black bile, two pairs of humors with opposite qualities. We recognize here the Pythagorean influence. Blood was said to originate in the heart, phlegm in the brain, yellow bile in the liver and black bile in the spleen.

It may seem queer that the spleen should have assumed the rank of a cardinal organ, since it is rather inconspicuous and systematic dissections were not performed in those days. The explanation may be that these theories were elaborated in malaria regions. Megalospleny is a symptom of chronic malaria, and these tremendously enlarged spleens could be palpated even more easily than the liver. Thus the spleen, located in the left part of the abdominal cavity, seemed to balance the liver on the right.

The theory of the four humors was further developed by Galen and still more by the Arabs, particularly by Avicenna in the early 11th century. It was a highly workable theory and explained a great deal. Each humor had elementary qualities. Thus blood was hot and moist like air; phlegm was cold and moist like water. Yellow bile was hot and dry like fire, and black bile was cold and dry like earth. Man was part of nature. Nature was constituted by the four elements, the human body by the four humors, and elements and humors had their elementary qualities in common. They formed the bridge between the microcosm and the macrocosm.

When the humors were normal in quantity and quality and well mixed so that the condition of *Eukrasia* prevailed, man was healthy. When, however, as a result of disturbances, one humor came to dominate in an abnormal way, the balance was upset, the mixture was bad, a *Dyskrasia* prevailed and the individual was sick. What then happened was that the organism, by virtue of its innate healing power which later was called the *vis medicatrix naturae,* endeavored to restore the balance. The humors which were considered crude in the beginning of the disease, underwent a process of ripening, a *coction;* and when they had matured, the faulty matter, the *materia peccans,* was driven out in the urine, the stools, the sputum or as pus. Whereupon the balance was restored and the patient cured. Or, if the disturbance was such that nature could not overcome it, the patient succumbed.

The very important practical consequence of these views was that the physician was taught to direct his entire treatment in such a way that it would assist the innate healing power of the body and to avoid whatever might possibly antagonize it. He did this by prescribing an appropriate diet, the effect of which could be enhanced by drugs. Or, in certain cases, he took recourse to the knife. By opening an abscess he helped nature to drive out the pus, thus shortening the process and saving the forces of the organism.

The theory of the elementary qualities permitted Galen in the 2nd century A. D. to develop an elaborate pharmacological system that was followed for almost fifteen hundred years.[1] The humors had elementary qualities, and since they determined the character of the diseases, these had also dominating qualities. Drugs, too like other objects of nature, had definite qualities, and thus a disease that was hot and moist was to be cured by drugs that were cold and dry. Galen differentiated between four groups of qualities in drugs, occurring in four degrees of intensity. His system was extremely popular in the Middle Ages, in Arabic as well as in Western medicine, because it gave the physician well defined instructions.

The theory of the four humors could also be used to explain the various constitutional types of men.[2] No two individuals are the same, to be sure, but one can distinguish certain groups. There are tall and short, fat and lean, intelligent and dumb, irascible and sullen individuals. It was observed in antiquity that certain physical and mental qualities occur in definite combinations. Stout persons are usually good-natured. The devil is never pictured as fat, for this would have made him a good devil. The humoral theory seemed to explain these differences. It was assumed that one of the four humors could slightly dominate *dia physin,* that is physiologically, without causing disease. Thus if the black bile, the *melaina chole* dominated, the individual belonged to the melancholic type which Aristotle described in the Problems.[3] It was a type to which many men of genius belonged, philosophers, statesmen, artists, but a somewhat unbalanced type which today we would call manic-depressive, people who sometimes are in high spirits and sometimes deeply depressed. Later these types were related to the planets. The melancholic man was the Saturnian man that Albrecht Dürer has pictured on his well-known woodcut.[4]

Similarly, it was assumed that the blood, the phlegm, and the yellow bile could dominate physiologically, and the Arabs described the sanguine, phlegmatic and choleric types. These views persisted for a long time, and it is impossible to understand Shakespeare's plays if one is not familiar with them.

I have discussed the theory of the four humors in such detail, because it had a most prolonged influence on medical thought, and because it illustrated most graphically the philosophic interpretation of disease. Every medical theory is based on observation and reasoning, and every period thinks with the concepts available at the time. The humoral theory was the result of many brilliant and correct observations. It was logical, explained many phenomena of health and disease, and gave valuable guidance to the medical practitioner. It was not scientific in our sense of the word: nobody had ever seen the black bile, and the qualities hot, cold, dry, moist were not physical concepts. Sea water was considered dry, pepper hot, while the rose was cold. Qualities were not measured but assumed logically on the ground of certain observations. There was science in antiquity, highly developed mathematics, physics, astronomy. Scientific experiments were made in biology too, but the scientific means were not available for an interpretation of health and disease, and the need for a comprehension of these phenomena was satisfied by philosophic speculation.

The theory of the four humors was by no means the only one in antiquity. As a matter of fact it was fully developed rather late and was much more influential in the Middle Ages than in antiquity. Other interpretations of disease were given. While the Hippocratic physicians considered the humors the most essential factors in the genesis of disease, others held the solid particles to be more important. Under the influence of the atomistic theories of Epicurus,

Asklepiades in the 1st century B. C. developed a new theory and laid the foundation for a new school. According to him, the human body was built of atoms, which joined to form the structural parts and were in constant motion in the pores of the organism. Health prevailed as long as the atoms were able to move freely; disease developed when the motion was disturbed. The disciples of Asklepiades, elaborating his doctrine, reduced the vital processes to two basic functions, namely, contraction and relaxation. They assumed that all solid parts had the faculty of contracting or relaxing. Disease was nothing else but abnormal contraction or relaxation in some part of the body. The theory led to a simple *method* of treatment, and the followers of this school were therefore called *Methodicists*. Some of the most brilliant physicians of antiquity belonged to it.

Philosophical skepticism had its repercussions in medicine also. A school of physicians sprang from Alexandria in the 3rd century B. C. which repudiated all attempts to interpret the nature of health and disease. They pointed out that the purpose of medicine was to cure sick people, and that doctors belonging to very different schools still produced the same results. They made experience their guide: their own and that of others as related in literature, and when experience was lacking they acted by analogy. There were excellent practitioners among these *Empiricists*.[5]

All these schools existed side by side for centuries. In the early Middle Ages Methodicism had a certain vogue, but from the 12th century on, when the Arabic literature became known to the West, the theory of the four humors dominated all others. It was at its height in the Renaissance when it experienced its first devastating attack. The attack came from Philip Theophrastus von Hohenheim who called himself Paracelsus (1493–1541).

The natural sciences had greatly progressed. The voyages of discovery had stimulated studies in geography and long distance navigation was setting new problems to physics and astronomy. New inventories were made of the animal and vegetable kingdoms, while the mining and the smelting of ore called for new chemical investigations. There was a general trend towards realism. People began to distrust the traditional authorities and wanted to see things for themselves. And they had the courage to trust their own eyes, even if what they saw contradicted the traditions.

Paracelsus was a physician, but he was also a scientist particularly well-versed in chemistry. He had worked in mines and smelters, and on his long peregrinations had accumulated a great deal of experience. The introduction of many chemical drugs was probably his greatest practical contribution to medicine. He was very much interested in such diseases as gout, arthritis, stone diseases that he called the tartaric diseases, and it struck him that there was a great deal of analogy between the physiological and pathological processes of the human body and the chemical reactions that he observed in his laboratory. Would it not be possible to explain the mechanism of disease in terms of chemistry? This could not be done on the traditional theory of the four humors, which he attacked most violently whenever he had an opportunity. Gradually, he developed his own theory whereby he made use of chemical concepts. There are humors, of course—nobody can deny their existence—but they do not play the part attributed to them by the Galenic school. What is important is that in every organ three principles can be found: the combustible, the volatile, and the incombustible which remains as an ash. He named these three principles symbolically *sulphur, mercury,* and *salt.* This gave him the chemical material that constituted the human body, but he needed an additional concept for the alchemist who used the material and effected the chemical reactions. He assumed the existence of a vital principle which he named *archaeus.*

Paracelsus was a Renaissance scientist. Dissatisfied with the traditional medical theories, he developed his own system. It was meant to be scientific, but actually, although concepts of science were used, it was a philosophic system and was just as speculative as the Greek systems had been.

Paracelsus was not satisfied with explaining the mechanism of disease. He wanted to know why and how man becomes sick. He discussed these problems in a book to which he gave the mysterious title *Volumen Paramirum*.[6] It deals with the five *entia,* the five spheres that determine man's life in health and disease.

The first is *ens astrale*. Every individual is born at a definite time, and the historical moment at which we live has a great influence on our physical life. Then there is *ens veneni,* which means that we all live in a given physical environment from which we derive matter and energy. But from nature come poisons also, and all the abnormal stimuli that cause disease. Everything that comes from nature is therefore good and evil, food, poison, and remedy. It is the *dosage* that determines the effect. The third sphere, *ens naturale,* means that all individuals are different. Each man is born with a nature of his own, and he thus to a large extent carries his destiny within himself. But man is also a spiritual being and from this, from the fourth sphere, *ens spirituale,* may also emanate causes of disease.

Such is the fourfold order under which man lives in the scheme of Paracelsus. If he is well adjusted to it, he is in good health; but from these four spheres may come diseases and man then returns to the normal condition in the fifth sphere, the sphere of God, *ens Dei*.

Paracelsus reveals himself as a scientist in search of a philosophy of medicine. He was not satisfied with treating patients but asked for the *how* and *why* of disease. He was a spiritualist and vitalist. His influence was felt after his death when his writings became known. Van Helmont and the *iatrochemists* of the 17th century looked to him as their ancestor. They all tried to explain life in health and disease in terms of chemistry, but basically they remained philosophers of nature. It was impossible to interpret physiology in chemical terms with any accuracy before Lavoisier had introduced quantitative methods into chemistry.

Lavoisier died in 1794 and the revolution of chemistry took place relatively late. Chemistry for a long time was burdened by a mystical heritage. Alchemy had sometimes exhibited the character of a religious movement in which the attraction and repulsion of chemical bodies assumed the value of symbols. Alchemists were seeking the elixir of youth and the *lapis philosophorum* with the help of which it should be possible to transmute one metal into another. It was tempting and easy to link up chemical with astrological views. Paracelsus had tried to set chemistry new tasks and to make it a scientific discipline, but his own mysticism misled many of his followers.

Conditions were different in physics, the foundation of which was mathematics. Galileo died in 1642 and physics was more than a century ahead of chemistry. In 1628 William Harvey, in describing the circulation of the blood, demonstrated that a difficult problem of physiology could be solved experimentally by applying principles of physics. We shall discuss his work in more detail in the following chapter. Harvey's discovery, once it was accepted, made a profound impression. If physics could explain the motion of the blood, it seemed very likely that it could also explain other physiological and even pathological processes.

Throughout the 17th century physicians were actively exploring the functions of life in health and disease in terms of physics. Descartes' philosophy influenced them very strongly. The trouble with these iatrophysicists or iatromechanists was that they were impatient. Harvey was a great man not only because he made a great discovery but also because he knew his own limitations. He solved one problem once and for all, and he had the courage to leave other problems unsolved. He explained only what he could demonstrate experimentally and was not afraid to admit that he had no answer for other questions. This makes him a true scientist.

Most of his followers were different. They endeavored to establish complete systems that would explain all phenomena of health and disease without any gap. When they spoke of the teeth as scissors that cut the food and millstones that grind it, they were not far from the truth because this was a simple function that could be verified easily. But when they spoke of the lungs as a pair of bellows, or of the intestines as being sieves, they were speaking allegorically and were indulging in speculation.

Thus the same happened with the iatrophysicists as with the iatrochemists. They used concepts of the new science, they made some contributions toward solving problems of minor detail, but basically their approach was philosophical and their systems were short-lived.

Medical science progressed very slowly and an infinity of problems was and still is left unsolved. This is very unsatisfactory, and therefore physicians at all times were inclined to supplement their scientific knowledge with philosophic speculation.

Every system of philosophy had repercussions in medicine, just as the experience of medicine and science had repercussions on philosophy. When we look at the development that took place in the last few centuries, we find that two basic approaches were constantly contending with each other. On one side were what we may broadly call the materialists. As science progressed it was found that the human body was built of the same elements that constitute inorganic nature. In 1828 the chemist Friedrich Wöhler was able to produce urea synthetically in the laboratory and without using the kidneys. He thus broke down the barrier between organic and inorganic chemistry and demonstrated that the organic compounds produced by the animal organism were not basically different from other compounds. More and more it became evident that many functions of life were physical processes or chemical reactions, and with increasing knowledge the borderline between physics and chemistry has been virtually eradicated.

This materialistic approach was extremely fertile. It was responsible for most of the progress thereafter achieved, and even deeply religious scientists when they entered their laboratories forgot their spiritualism and conducted their researches along materialistic lines. Many problems of physiology and pathology were elucidated in this way, but one problem remained unsolved, the problem of life itself. How did dead food become living substance? How did an organism develop from a fertilized ovum? What force permitted cells to regenerate lost tissue?

There is no reason why we should be impatient. Science is still very young. Two hundred years ago electricity was hardly known: today we not only make extensive use of it, but it has revolutionized our views on the structure of matter. One hundred years ago organic chemistry was in its very beginnings and today we are not only familiar with but can also synthesize an endless number of organic substances. Chemistry, from the gross chemistry it was, is becoming microchemistry; and we begin to see the effects of a substance in infinitely small quantities, even of single molecules. Recent studies on the crystallization of disease viruses are opening up new horizons. There really is no reason why it should not some day be possible to solve the problem of life scientifically.

People, however, have at all times been impatient and have created concepts to explain what their knowledge failed to account for. Aristotle distinguished between natural bodies that possess life and those that do not. By life he meant the power of self-nourishment and of independent growth and decay. He assumed that a body was living because it was endowed with a principle which he called psyche or soul. He distinguished various forms of soul: the vegetative soul responsible for nutrition and reproduction, the animal soul directing motion and sensibility, and the rational soul peculiar to man and making him a conscious and intellectual being. He was a vitalist and in addition a teleologist, because he assumed that every part of the body was made for a certain end, every organ for a separate function, and the body as a whole for the soul. Similarly Galen and his followers believed in vital principles which they called spirits.

When the authority of Aristotle and Galen waned and mechanistic views dominated biology, vitalism was revived.[7] In 1748 La Mettrie published *L'Homme Machine,* a book that interpreted the body as a machine in the crudest possible fashion. In 1759 Caspar Friedrich Wolff wrote a *Theoria Generationis* in which he attacked the mechanists. He believed in a *vis essentialis* that developed the organism and produced and moved the machine of the body. In 1789 vitalism reached a peak with J. F. Blumenbach's treatise *Über den Bildungstrieb.* Blumenbach added to the three traditional vital forces, namely, contractibility, irritability and sensibility, a fourth one, the *nisus formativus,* the formative impulse which produces the organic form and regenerates it after mutilations.

Vitalism found a fertile soil in Germany in the early 19th century, the period of romanticism and *Naturphilosophie* when medicine indulged in regular orgies of philosophical speculation. While the French physicians were studying diseases at the bedside of patients and were performing autopsies in their laboratories, the German physicians sat at their desks and wrote treatises on the nature of disease and of the world at large. There is no point in reviewing their absurd theories. The titles of a few books published at that time reflect the spirit in which they were written: [8]

Comparative idealist pathology, an attempt to present the diseases as relapses of the idea of life to lower, normal degrees of life.
Ideas about the construction of disease.
Forebodings of a general natural history of diseases.
A system of tellurism.
On the internal structure of the healing art.

Preliminary studies on a philosophical history of medicine as the
    safest foundation for the present reform of this science.
Paieon or popular philosophy of medicine and its history.
Axioms from the metaphysics of nature applied to chemical and
    medical subjects.
A dualistic system of medicine, or doctrine of the antitheses in the
    forces of the living animal organism.[9]

These books were written while Laennec in France published
his classical treatise on auscultation and the diseases of the chest.
Germany emerged from this nightmare in the eighteen-forties and
with Helmholtz medicine took a sharp turn to the laboratory.
German medicine never had a steady and straight-forward development. It always went from one extreme to the other.[10] This
was at the same time its weakness and its strength. What Albrecht
von Haller once said of the English applies much more to the
Germans: "Whatever this people undertakes, it brings to perfection, the good as well as the evil." [11]

After a period of philosophical idealism and unrestrained speculation, Germany had a period of philosophical materialism with
Feuerbach, Marx, Engels, Vogt, Büchner. Medicine became extremely scientific and soon had a leading position in the world. The
pendulum swung back. Hans Driesch, von Uexküll and others
developed a neo-vitalism. Neo-Hippocratism, neo-Paracelsism and
other similar, basically romantic and mystic movements came to
the fore. They were the precursors of Hitlerism. Germany is again
engulfed in a wave of mysticism, but she will emerge from it as
she has emerged in the past, and it is not difficult to guess what
direction the reaction will take.

History teaches us that the political philosophy of a nation
exerts a great influence on its science. Medicine is a rational subject and therefore cannot flourish when the underlying philosophy
is mystical, as was the case in the Middle Ages, in the period of
German romanticism, and now again under Fascism. What saved

medicine from collapse in Fascist countries was their imperialistic program. Modern war is a highly scientific matter and calls upon all the resources of medical science. The necessity of preparing for total war has to a certain extent kept Fascist medicine earthbound and has prevented it from losing itself in mystical speculations.

Where, on the other hand, the underlying philosophy is rational medical science has the best possible opportunity. This is the case in the United States, a country built on the foundation of 18th century rationalism. It is also the case in the Soviet Union where for the first time in history an attempt is being made to organize society in all its aspects along scientific lines.

The physician should not be afraid to engage in philosophical studies. If he wants to be more than a narrow specialist, he must look at medicine from a wide perspective and must be aware of the place that medicine takes in our body of knowledge. If he is a true scientist, his thought will be disciplined and he will not lose himself in unrestrained speculation.

NOTES

1. Henry E. Sigerist, *Studien und Texte zur frühmittelalterlichen Rezeptliteratur,* Leipzig, 1923, pp. 11–16.
2. Henry E. Sigerist, Wandlungen des Konstitutionsbegriffs, *Internat. ärztlicher Fortbildungskursus, 1928,* (*Karlsbader ärztliche Vorträge,* Band 10) Jena, 1929, pp. 97–108.
3. XXX, 1.
4. E. Panofsky and F. Saxl, *Dürers "Melencolia I,"* Leipzig, Berlin, 1923.
5. Karl Deichgräber, *Die griechische Empirikerschule,* Berlin, 1930.
6. Henry E. Sigerist, Paracelsus in the Light of 400 Years, *The March of Medicine,* New York, Columbia University Press, 1941, pp. 38–40.
7. See Hans Driesch, *Geschichte des Vitalismus,* Leipzig, 1922.
8. See Ernst Hirschfeld, Romantische Medizin, *Kyklos,* 1930, vol. 3, pp. 1–89 with

good bibliography. See also Martin Heun, *Die medizinische Zeitschriftenliteratur der Romantik*, Diss. Leipzig, 1931.

9. Full titles in Hirschfeld, *l.c.*

10. Henry E. Sigerist, Heilkunde in: *Sachwörterbuch der Deutschkunde*, Berlin, 1930.

11. *Albrecht Hallers Tagebücher seiner Reisen . . . 1723–1727*, herausgegeben von Ludwig Hirzel, Leipzig, 1883, p. 139.

CHAPTER VIII

Disease and Science

IN THE LAST two chapters we discussed the religious and philosophical interpretations of disease. The scientific approach was a great step forward in that it gave the physician a solid foundation upon which to build. Disease could be interpreted logically in philosophical terms in a way that would satisfy the inquisitive mind, but when it came to testing philosophic theory in actual practice the physician was often left in the lurch. Medicine is a *techne*, a craft. The physician's task is not to interpret the world in which he lives but to protect and restore the health of his fellow men. He must have a theory to correlate the diversity of phenomena, but the theory must be applicable to practice. It must give the physician guidance and must make him more efficient in the treatment of patients.

In the 17th century the school of the iatrophysicists reached its peak in Giorgio Baglivi. Iatrophysics provided him with a theory that satisfied his need for causality. He freely confessed, however, that when it came to treating the sick, he followed the principles of Hippocrates—principles based on a totally different doctrine. In other words, Baglivi's theory was worthless to him as a physician. Whenever there was such a rift between theory and practice, medicine did not progress and all that physicians could do was to act on the basis of experience.

There is no doubt that experience means a great deal in medicine. Pharmacological theories changed, but castor-oil was used

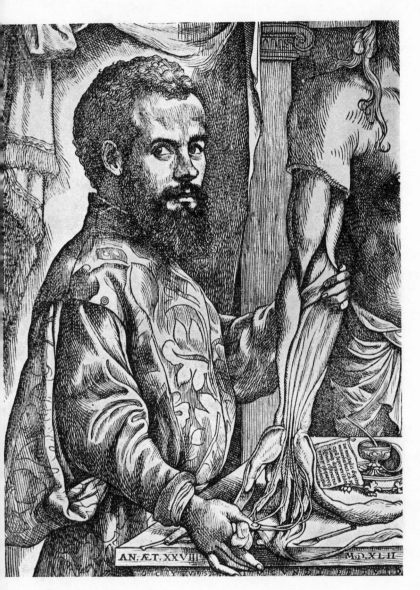

25. ANDREAS VESALIUS (1514–1564). The founder of modern anatomy.

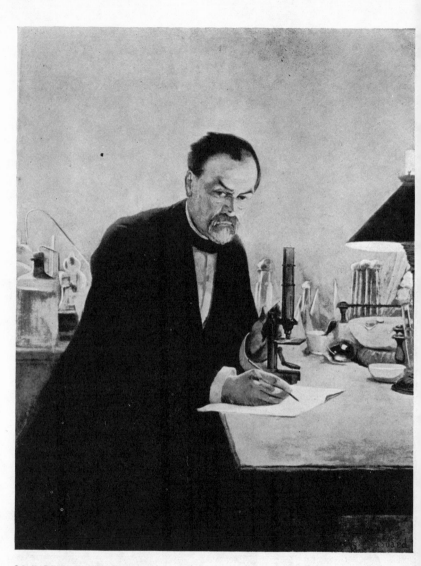

26. LOUIS PASTEUR (1822–1895). (After the painting of L. Fournier.)

effectively for thousands of years. Cinchona and fox-glove were popular remedies and were used by physicians empirically. The moment, however, that medicine had a scientific pharmacological theory it was not only able to explain the effect of accepted drugs but also to find new ones systematically. Similarly, experience taught that malaria occurred in the vicinity of swamps. The theory was that in the summer and autumn swamps developed pernicious exhalations. It was a logical assumption and not a scientific fact, because nobody had ever been able to capture or analyze these exhalations. The theory was wrong, yet it was helpful. On the basis of it, the popes from the 16th to the 18th centuries drained parts of the Pontine marshes with good results. The moment, however, the scientific fact was established that malaria is caused by a microorganism transmitted by mosquitoes, the disease could be combated much more systematically.

The development of medical science was very slow because it depended upon the development of the other sciences and was part of the establishment of what Charles Singer has very justly called the *mechanical world*.[1] One step was taken after another, very slowly, and at no time was medical science able to provide a complete, logically integrated system as the ancient theories had done. Many interrogation marks have survived to our own day, but every scientific advance was a permanent gain which brought medicine closer to its goal.

Disease manifests itself in disturbed function. Hence it was necessary to investigate normal function before it became possible to establish a new, a scientific pathology. In other words, pathology had to be preceded by a new physiology. Since function is nothing else than the vital manifestation of the organs, the new physiology could not develop before the foundations of a new anatomy had been laid. This took place at the time of the Renaissance, which thus marks the beginning of a new era in medicine.

Anatomy, of course, had existed long before the Renaissance. Whoever opened an animal for culinary or sacrificial purposes possessed a certain anatomical knowledge. The Greeks had explored the structure of the animal organism just as they had investigated other objects of nature. They had dissected a great variety of animals and, in Alexandria for a while, also human cadavers. According to tradition they had even performed vivisections on criminals. Greek anatomy, however, as it had been transmitted through the Middle Ages, was largely animal anatomy.

From the beginning of the 14th century, human cadavers were dissected publicly in the medical schools of the universities. These dissections were performed not for purposes of research but as demonstrations. The faith in traditional authorities was still unshaken, and it was assumed that ancient anatomy could not be improved. Conditions changed toward the end of the 15th and in the 16th century with growing skepticism, when the development of a new attitude led to an open revolt against the established authorities. It was found that ancient anatomy described the structure of animals, not that of man, who was the center of the humanists' interest. Him they wanted to know, and since traditions failed them, they had to undertake the work of exploration themselves. Artists and physicians, men like Leonardo da Vinci and Andreas Vesalius went ahead, dissected body after body, and described their findings with pen and pencil.

A new descriptive human anatomy was founded. In 1543 Vesalius published in Basle his "Seven Books on the Structure of the Human Body"—*De Corporis Humani Fabrica Libri Septem.* Vesalius was well aware that he had made an important contribution, but the significance of his book was infinitely greater than he could possibly realize. It not only gave a more complete and more accurate picture of the human body than any previous work, but was also to become the corner-stone of a new medicine—a scientific medicine based on anatomy.

Throughout the 16th century anatomical research was carried out vigorously, and the more intimately the structure of the body became known, the more pronounced the desire was to explore the purpose and function of the organs. The ancient physiological theories explained the phenomena of life, but more and more physicians were thinking in terms of anatomy, looking at the body as a machine of which every organ was a part. A theory that was anatomically impossible was no longer considered satisfactory. From a static subject anatomy gradually became a dynamic science—*anatomia animata*.

The turning point had come for physiology when Harvey in 1628 described the circulation of the blood.[2] In order to understand the full significance of his discovery we must remember what traditional views were held about the motion of the blood. The starting point of all physiology was the elementary observation that there are substances in nature such as food and air that are necessary for life. Without food an organism starves to death and without air it suffocates. But it was also found that there is a substance in the human body that must be necessary for life because it occurs throughout the organism, namely, blood that escapes from every wound. Physiology began with speculations about the relationship between these substances.

The theory that dominated physiology before Harvey was derived from Galen, who had taught that food was digested in the stomach, moved to the intestines, when it passed through the veins into the liver. In the liver food was turned into blood and was impregnated with the natural spirit, a principle that was believed to regulate what we now call the vegetative functions of the body. Part of this dark liver blood streamed into the entire organism, while one part went through the vena cava into the right ventricle of the heart where a further division took place. One portion of this blood went to the lungs, where it unloaded waste materials of the body. This explained why the air breathed out was different from the air breathed in. Another portion of the blood went through the septum of the heart into the left ventricle where it was mixed with air that came from the lungs in the pulmonary vein. This mixture of air and blood generated the vital spirit that controlled the animal functions. It also generated the body heat which was regulated by respiration. This explained why we breathe more frequently when the body is too hot as a result of work or fever. From the left side of the heart the blood—a light blood different from that of the liver—streamed through the arteries into the organism, and one portion went to the brain where it was charged with the animal spirit that controlled the nervous functions.

This was a very comprehensive theory which explained logically the relationship between food, blood, and air, and provided a system that appeared invulnerable. It was qualitative and was derived from very correct observations by means of speculation.

Harvey's approach was different. He was an anatomist and had dissected not just human bodies but a variety of animals, dead and alive. Aristotelian by tradition, he was a contemporary of Galileo and thought in terms of mechanics. He found the septum of the heart to be a solid muscle through which blood could not possibly pass. He saw that the systole, the contraction of the heart, was the active element of its motion, and that with every contraction it ejected blood into the arteries. And then Harvey asked himself one question, whose very phrasing marked a new departure. He asked *how much* blood left the heart with every contraction, and he found that it was about two ounces. In other words, with a heartbeat of 72 a minute the amount of blood ejected from the heart in one hour was 72 x 60 x 2 or 8,640 ounces, which is over three times the body weight. Harvey concluded that the blood ejected from the heart through the arteries returned to it through the veins in a circulatory motion. This was a logical conclusion, and through a series of experiments Harvey was able to prove scientifically that it was correct.

Harvey's theory had one important gap. The capillaries were not known as yet, and in assuming that there must be a passage for the blood from the arteries to the veins Harvey was making use of a hypothesis. He could do it safely because his theory was based on mathematical evidence. As a matter of fact the capillaries were discovered a few decades later by Malpighi with the help of the microscope.

Harvey's theory was much less complete than that of Galen. It did not explain the relation between food and blood nor the function of respiration. He limited himself to the solution of one problem that he could attack experimentally and mathematically. He solved it once and for all, leaving the solution of other problems to further research. This is the procedure of science.

Anatomy and physiology did not yet constitute a new system of medicine. In the 17th century disease was still interpreted in the traditional, that is philosophical, way even when physicians used concepts of the new science. The development of anatomy and physiology, however, by leading to a more intimate knowledge of structure and function of the body gradually permitted a scientific approach to the problem of disease. The next great step was taken when Morgagni in 1761 published his "Five Books on the Seats and Causes of Diseases, Investigated Anatomically"—*De Sedibus et Causis Morborum per Anatomen Indagatis.*

In dissecting the bodies of people who had died from disease, the anatomists often found abnormal conditions such as adhesions, ulcers, tumors, or stones. Morgagni set out to correlate these findings with the symptoms of disease observed during an individual's fatal illness. He established the method of medical investigation that has been used very successfully ever since, namely, the comparison of data of the clinical case history and of the autopsy report. He came to the conclusion that disease can be localized, that it has a seat, that it resides in the organs. The diseased organs are different in their structure from normal organs, and since their structure is different their function is different also; this abnormal function causes what appears as disease symptoms. The character of the anatomical lesion determines the kind of disease prevailing.

Later, in the early 19th century, diseases were traced back to the tissues (Bichat), and still later, in 1858, to the cells (Virchow).

Like physiology, pathology had become anatomical and this new approach, although it left many problems unsolved, yet marked a great progress. Disease entities could now be defined much more sharply. Diseases such as pneumonia, gastric ulcer, cirrhosis of the liver, cancer of the uterus were characterized not merely by a group of clinical symptoms but by typical anatomical changes. Pathological anatomy, in addition to its great scientific interest, had tremendous practical consequences. If the physician was able to find out what anatomical changes had occurred in a patient, he could make a much more accurate diagnosis of the disease than in the past. And correct diagnosis gave him valuable leads as to the prognosis, particularly after the statistical method had been widely applied to the clinical field. The diagnosis also largely determined the treatment that was to be followed.

This new attitude was responsible for the development of such methods of physical diagnostics as percussion and auscultation. By knocking on the thorax, by listening to the heart-beat and the respiratory murmurs, the physician could form an opinion on the anatomical condition of these organs. Ingenious instruments were invented, such as the ophthalmoscope and the laryngoscope, that permitted the physician to look into the organs and see the changes directly. Electric bulbs and mirrors were introduced into all cavities of the body, and the physician's eye could penetrate into bronchi, stomach, duodenum, bladder and rectum. The triumph in this development was the application of the X-rays to diagnostic purposes. The X-rays made almost all parts of the human body accessible to the eye. Anatomical changes could be seen and recorded in photography.

When we look at the development of scientific medicine from the Renaissance on, we can see that anatomy was taking a central position in the new system. The anatomical method had invaded physiology in the 17th century, pathology in the 18th, clinical medicine in the early 19th century. There was only one field of medicine that had not yet been touched by this new approach, namely, therapy. The treatment of diseases was still following traditional lines and had progressed very little. A few effective new drugs had been introduced empirically, but as a whole the treatment of disease in the early 19th century was hardly more advanced than in Hippocratic days. The famous Viennese school was renowned for its therapeutic nihilism, and doctors were said to be interested in a patient only twice: when they made the diagnosis and when they performed the autopsy.

It was perfectly obvious that an anatomical pathology would call for an anatomical therapy, and this explains the tremendous development that surgery took from the middle of the 19th century on. Surgery was a craft. From antiquity it had developed slowly but steadily, benefiting from every anatomical and technical advance. As a matter of fact, the professor of surgery and the professor of anatomy were usually one and the same man. In the early 19th century surgery was still limited to a small number of classical operations and was applied when internal treatment was impossible or gave no result. However, once physicians conceived of disease in terms of anatomy, their attitude towards surgery changed. Surgery was no longer a last refuge but assumed a primary position in therapy. By cutting out an ulcer or a tumor the surgeon was presumably removing the disease itself and was thus correcting the anatomy of the organ. This changed attitude towards surgery explains why the two chief obstacles that had impeded the progress of surgery—pain and secondary infection—were overcome through the introduction of general anaesthesia and antisepsis. From a frequently despised craftsman the surgeon became the most spectacularly effective and therefore the most popular medical specialist.

Even pharmacology became, towards the end of the 19th century, anatomical to a certain extent. Drugs were no longer given merely on the basis of experience but because it had been found that certain chemical compounds had a well-defined affinity to particular cells of the human body. In giving a drug the physician was aiming at definite organs or tissues.

After having conquered one field of medicine after another, the anatomical cycle had come to an end. Anatomy still is and will remain the foundation of medicine, and anatomical considerations will always play an important part, but today we think primarily in terms of function and we find ourselves in the midst of a new, a physiological cycle.

Pathological anatomy was able to explain a great deal. It showed what changes occurred in the lungs in a case of pneumonia, and how these changes determined the symptoms of the disease. But it did not explain what causes pneumonia.

The acute infectious, and especially the epidemic diseases, had always attracted the people's attention in a particular way. Other diseases could be understood as the result of faulty diet or the wrong mode of living of an individual. But in the case of epidemics large groups of very different people, men and women, young and old, strong and weak were equally attacked by the same disease. Once the religious interpretation was discarded, physicians were looking for natural causes and they made the environment of man, particularly cosmic, telluric and atmospheric conditions, responsible for the disease. When a certain epidemic constitution prevailed in nature, people exposed to it fell sick.

But then it was also seen that epidemic diseases spread by contact from man to man. This was particularly evident in the epidemics of plague. Whoever touched a sick man or even his clothes was apt to contract the disease himself. The conclusion from such observations was that there must be a substance that causes the disease, a matter that is found in the sick, in his excretions and on the objects of his immediate environment. Mediaeval epidemiological measures were intended to destroy that substance. But what was its nature?

The phenomenon of parasitism was well known from earliest antiquity. Intestinal worms were frequent in the East and could be seen in human and animal discharges. In the 17th century the microscope opened up a new world of infinitely small organisms, too small to be perceived by the unaided eye, the infusoria and even bacteria that Leeuwenhoek found on his own tongue. Could it be that the infectious substance was animated and consisted of such tiny animalcules? The idea was in the air for several centuries.

In 1840 the German anatomist Jacob Henle published a pathological treatise of which the first section, *On Miasmata and Contagia,* has become a classic.[3] Henle did not see the microorganisms that cause disease, but he deduced that the pathogenic matter must be animated and the logic of his argumentation was irresistible. In those days the traditional distinction was still made between *miasma* and *contagium.* Miasma was the disease substance that invaded an organism from the outside nature. Malaria was the prototype of a miasmatic disease that was always acquired from outside and never by direct contact with the sick. Contagium, on the other hand, designated the disease substance that was believed to be generated in the sick organism and spread the disease by contact. Syphilis was a contagious disease because it was acquired by contact exclusively. Most epidemic diseases, however, were considered miasmatic-contagious, that is, they could be acquired from outside but also by contact.

If miasma and contagium can cause the same disease, Henle argued, they must be identical. And he further concluded that they must be not only organic but also animated, because a dead substance would be used up in the patient, while the disease matter, on the contrary, grew and multiplied in the sick body after the manner of a parasite. Such substances were known. In 1835 Cagniard de Latour had demonstrated that yeast, which causes alcoholic fermentation, is not a dead substance but a fungus, and it became obvious that the life activity of such a fungus could cause great chemical changes.

This is where Pasteur's work began twenty years later. In studying various types of fermentation, he found that other fungi, the *bacteria,* had effects similar to that of yeast. He could demonstrate the ubiquity of bacteria and he found that many of them were pathogenic, that they caused diseases by invading the organism and living on it as parasites. In 1876 Robert Koch described the life-cycle of the bacterium that was responsible for the anthrax disease. There could no longer be any doubt concerning the nature of the contagium, and one microorganism after another was found to be the specific cause of certain diseases.

Bacteriology did not solve all problems of infectious diseases, and it was found that some were caused by still smaller agents that pass the finest filters, the so-called *viruses.* These consist of large protein molecules and although they still present many unsolved problems, it has been possible to attack many virus diseases successfully.

The consequences of all these discoveries were tremendous. Once the immediate cause of contagious diseases was known, it became possible to combat them at the root. Hygiene and public health were put on a new foundation. Surgery was freed from the nightmare of secondary infection. With vaccines and serums it became possible to immunize people against an increasing number

174

of diseases. In our last chapter we shall discuss in more detail the effect of these discoveries on the people's health.

We have already mentioned that chemistry had its great revolution towards the end of the 18th century when it became a quantitative science. This was only yesterday, and in the short period of 150 years chemistry, or rather physico-chemistry, has revolutionized our life. For thousands of years mankind depended for the satisfaction of some of its basic needs on the raw materials provided by nature and on the products of agriculture. Today we can make fertilizers with the nitrogen of the air. We no longer depend on natural deposits of oil but can prepare gasoline synthetically. We can make rubber from alcohol, oil and other complex chemicals. We produce fibers for textiles in the laboratory. Alloys and plastics can be made that are not mere *ersatz* for natural products but new man-made materials, superior in many ways to those of nature. A new technology has arisen and no limit is set to the physico-chemist's endeavors.

In biology chemistry has opened up new fields of physiology and pathology, making it possible to investigate the metabolism of the healthy and sick organism. Tests have been devised that permit us to form an opinion on the functional conditions of various organs. Nutrition, empirical in the past, has become a science through biochemistry, which has also explained the cause and mechanism of many very obscure diseases associated with the function of hormones and vitamins. But biochemistry has done much more than explain diseases: it has provided new means for their prevention and cure.

Chemistry finally became the core of a new pharmacology which investigated the action of chemical compounds on the normal and diseased organism. Pharmacology was able to discover affinities between certain parts of the body and certain chemical groups, and we can now produce systematically such chemical bodies as will have the desired effect.

At the present moment chemotherapy is yielding impressive results. Bacteriology had explained the cause of infectious diseases and given important methods for the protection of individuals. But when a disease had taken hold of a person, medicine was in many cases still helpless and thousands of people died every year from such diseases as pneumonia, meningitis or puerperal fever. In the beginning of our century Paul Ehrlich began a systematic search for chemical bodies that would kill bacteria without killing their host. In 1910 he produced *salvarsan,* which proved to be highly effective against a certain group of protozoa such as spirochetes and trypanosomes. But bacteria, our chief enemies, once they were firmly entrenched in the body seemed resistant against chemicals—until Gerhard Domagk discovered the action of the drug prontosil, later to be developed and known as sulfanilamide. This was in 1935, only yesterday, and in the last few years dozens of highly effective sulfadrugs have been prepared. There is every hope that more such drugs will be found in the very near future.

Bacteriology and chemistry became the chief weapons against infectious diseases, and from biochemistry we may expect the solution of many more pathological problems. Now that the acute diseases of childhood and youth have receded and more people are becoming old, the chronic diseases of maturity and old age— the wear-and-tear diseases—are in the foreground. Diseases of heart and circulation are the chief causes of death in the United States. We know a good deal about them but not enough. If biochemistry can elucidate their finer mechanism—and there is no reason why it could not—we may be able to prevent or at least to postpone them.

Cancer is still an unsolved problem. Its incidence has increased in proportion to the aging of the population. Although many early cases can be cured through surgical operations, X-ray and radium, yet a large-scale attack is impossible unless its cause and patho-genesis are known. Biochemistry may solve this problem also, un-less we are faced with a biological principle that still escapes us. It is extremely difficult to understand the biology of the cancer cell because it reacts differently from all other cells. In a differen-tiated organism the cells form a social community. They are special-ized and cooperate in a perfect way. The cancer cell is asocial. It goes its own ways, has its own metabolism, thrives at the expense of the organism like a parasite, destroys it and in so doing destroys itself. This is against all the rules and therefore is difficult to con-ceive.

When we look at the development of medical science, we must admit that the progress achieved in the last hundred years has been stupendous. It was in line with the development of the other sci-ences, taking advantage of every discovery made in physics, chem-istry or biology. The progress has been a steady one, and if we want to realize what has been achieved in the last few decades all we have to do is to read the first edition of Osler's textbook pub-lished in 1892 [4] and compare it with our present knowledge. We must not forget, however, that the advances of the last hundred years would have been impossible without the work of the cen-turies that preceded them. They represented the culminating point of a long and arduous development.

One hundred years ago there were only a few centers of medi-cal research. Today the work is carried on all over the world by tens of thousands of scientists. Millions are spent every year for research. There is a great amount of waste in this field as in our entire economy; there is lack of planning, lack of coordination, but the basis is so broad and the intelligence and energy spent on the task are so great that we may expect many more results.

The scientific interpretation of disease is still very young. We still have enormous gaps, and we know that the truth of today may appear as an error tomorrow. Yet we may face the future with confidence because we fill the gaps of our knowledge not with religious dreams or philosophical speculations but with scientific facts. And when we make use of working hypotheses, as we have to do all the time, we know that they are assumptions and we are ready to discard them whenever new facts warrant it.

Valuations and interpretations of scientific facts will undoubtedly change in the course of time. Factors that seem essential today may be considered secondary tomorrow. It may be found that the constitutional element is more important in the genesis of tuberculosis than the bacillus, but nevertheless the fact will remain that there is no tuberculosis without bacilli.

Our present theory of disease is still very primitive and new theories will certainly be elaborated in the course of time. We shall have new perspectives once we know more about the structure of matter, the physicochemistry of organic life and the nature of the nervous impulse, but whatever theory will be developed, it will make use of our present scientific facts.

The religious interpretation of disease is a dream; the philosophical interpretation is a painting that you relegate to the attic when you weary of it. But the scientific interpretation is a building of which every stone can be used for further construction.

Young as medical science is, it permits us to be very optimistic as to the future. And the ultimate goal of medicine, the eradication of disease, distant as it may be, is no longer Utopian.

NOTES

1. *A Short History of Science to the Nineteenth Century,* Oxford, 1941.
2. William Harvey, *Exercitatio Anatomica de Motu Cordis et Sanguinis in Ani-*

malibus. An English Translation with Annotations by Chauncey D. Leake. Baltimore, Md. and Springfield, Ill., Charles C. Thomas, 1931.

3. Jacob Henle, *On Miasmata and Contagia.* Translated by George Rosen. Baltimore, The Johns Hopkins Press, 1938.

4. William Osler, *The Principles and Practice of Medicine.* New York, D. Appleton and Co., 1892.

CHAPTER IX

Disease and Literature

THE WRITING of history is an artistic process. The historian is a member of the society in which he lives, sharing its hopes and fears, its aspirations and frustrations. Driven by a burning interest, by an overpowering urge, he sets out to consult the past— not the past at large, but a certain period, a sequence of events, personalities or problems. He wants to know what things were like, and to this end he assembles all the documents he can find. They become sources to him; he questions them, makes them talk, tries to understand and interpret them. Gradually a period, events, people of the past long dead become alive to him, an experience which he wants to share with others through the living word and in literary form. He recreates the past and by so doing makes the writing of history an artistic process.

The writer Émile Zola once defined art as "la nature vue par un tempérament," nature seen through the medium of a human mind. In the same way we could define history as the past seen through the medium of a human mind. Just as the artist communicates to others what he saw and felt, the historian transmits his experience. And this experience may be stirring and may drive people to action. Through the historian's work unconscious developments and trends acquire a new significance: people become aware of them, and this awareness may determine the course of their actions. This is why history, the picture we have of our past, is never dead

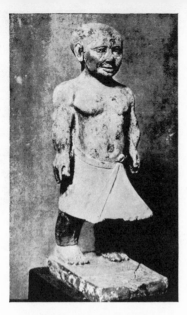

27. ACHONDROPLASIA.
The dwarf Chnoum-Hotep,
ca. 2700 B.C. (Cairo Museum.)

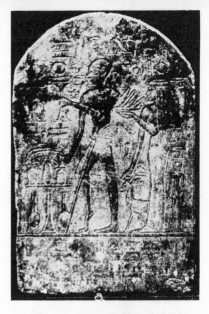

28. POLIOMYELITIS (?) The
priest Ruma, XVIIIth dynasty.
(Carlsberg Glyptothek, Copenhagen.)

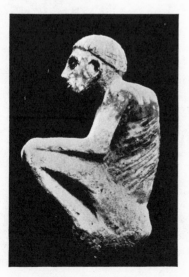

29. POTT'S DISEASE. An
Egyptian statuette of before

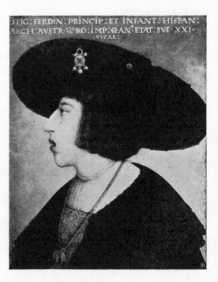

30. ADENOIDS. Ferdinand of
Spain, painted by Lucas of Leyden.

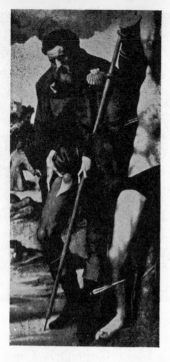

31. ST. ROCH, WITH PLAGUE BUBO. (Painting by Francesco Carotto, 1528.)

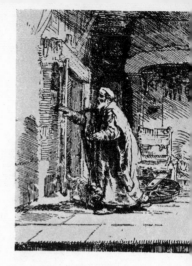

32. THE BLIND TOBIAS. (Etching by Rembrandt.)

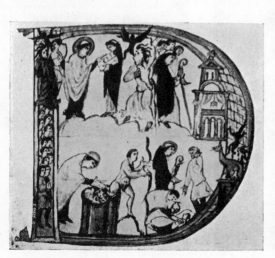

33. EXORCISING DEMONS. (Bibliothèque Nationale M.S.

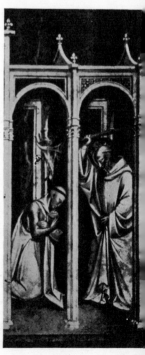

34. ST. BENEDICT EXORCIS-ING A DEMON BY FLOGGING

but, on the contrary, one of the most powerful driving forces of life.

From this also it results that the writing of history is a highly responsible task. The historian must submit to the iron discipline imposed upon him by the methods of historical research. They set sharp limits to his interpretations and forbid him to ascribe to an individual either actions or words unless he has documentary evidence for them. If he has to describe a case of illness, he must do so on the basis of records. The picture he gives of the past must be true, for only true history is fertile; faked history, written uncritically, or frivolously, or for purposes of propaganda is always destructive.[1] At this moment we are witnessing the distortion of minds and its fatal results created by political philosophies based on and justified by untrue historical considerations.

The poet, the novelist, and the dramatist also recreate aspects of the world. They too must be true if they want to be persuasive, but they enjoy much more freedom than the historian. They may create people, while the historian can only recreate them.

The writer always draws from his own experience, setting down what he has seen, what he has felt or thought. He has seen sickness, has observed that a serious illness may be the turning point in a man's life. He has experienced illness himself, for everybody has been afflicted by it at some time or other. Many great writers have suffered from tuberculosis: Shelley, Keats, Walt Whitman, Molière, Mérimée, Chekhov, Dostoevski, to mention only a few.[2] To some, like Schiller, it was a handicap which they struggled to overcome. To others, like Marie Bashkirtseff, it was the central experience of their lives which determined the character of their writings.

The number of physicians who became well-known writers of poetry, fiction, or drama is not small. It includes men like Haller, Chekhov, Schnitzler, Duhamel, Weir Mitchell, John Rathbone

Oliver, A. J. Cronin and many others. What could be more natural for them than to present medical problems or to use as motives disease and the suffering caused by it?

For all these reasons it is perfectly obvious that we should find descriptions of sick people and of diseases in an endless number of literary works from remote antiquity to our days, and it cannot be our purpose to catalogue them. Besides, the literature available on the subject is quite extensive because most classics have been read by cultivated physicians with pencil in hand. They have abstracted passages of medical interest and have written papers and monographs about them.[3] Or they have examined the diseases from which literary men suffered and how their work was affected.[4] In this brief chapter we must limit ourselves to a few general considerations on the subject and shall discuss particularly why a writer introduces disease into his work and how he pictures it.

Illness, in general, is not a good literary subject. In high school we had to write compositions on personal experiences, and our teacher used to warn us not to write about our measles or whooping cough or scarlet fever. He said that such an illness, of course, was an important experience to us but that a detailed description of it would be boring and of no interest to others. It was, moreover, unoriginal since thousands of other children had had the same experience.

This was good advice, and indeed outside the naturalist school that we shall discuss presently, writers as a rule describe cases of illness briefly and in general terms without the repulsive details —bleedings, diarrhoeas, vomitings—connected with many diseases. It is not the disease itself, but the effect it has on an individual's life that interests the writer.

In Tolstoi's great novel *Anna Karenina* the heroine after having given birth to her lover's child suffers from puerperal fever, and her illness marks a climax and turning point in the narrative. The disease is described in very general terms yet unmistakably. It is not the symptoms that count but the fact that Anna is going to die. She has broken the code of her society, has indulged in illicit love; her husband wants to divorce her, her lover is thrown out of his career; social ostracism will be her fate. Then she gives birth to the child, is taken sick and is going to die. In the face of death, the two men who love her, husband and lover, meet and shake hands with each other. The husband forgives her, the lover goes home and shoots himself. This could have ended the story, but the fact that it does not end makes it so great a novel. Anna recovers against expectation, the attempted suicide failed, life goes on. Anna and her lover escape by going abroad until, after a short period of bliss, life becomes intolerable to her and she kills herself.

In the same novel Tolstoi has used disease very cleverly in order to accentuate a situation. After Anna has killed herself, her lover in despair is going to war. He is waiting on the platform of a railroad station for a train to leave and at the same time he is suffering from an excruciating toothache. This may seem trivial, yet by adding the physical pain to the mental torment in which Vronski finds himself the intolerable situation is accentuated as forcefully as could be.

In a similar way disease is used in a great many novels, either in the evolution of the plot or in order to characterize a given situation. Since the novelist is not a medical man and since he is writing for laymen, he does not describe rare diseases known only to specialists but rather those with which everybody is familiar. The choice is determined primarily by two factors, the time at which a writer lives and the purpose to be attained.

In the 13th century Hartmann von Aue in his novel *Armer Heinrich* made his hero a leper in order to picture the self-sacrificing love of a young girl for her lord. This was the logical thing to do in the Middle Ages but would be out of place today, when leprosy has practically disappeared from the Western world.

Hans Pfitzner revived the subject in an opera in 1895 and Gerhard Hauptmann in a drama in 1902, but this was pure romanticism which consciously used mediaeval subjects on account of their human values. In a modern realistic novel a different condition would be chosen, as in Henry Bellamann's *Kings Row* where the self-sacrificing devotion of a woman to the man she loves and marries is illustrated by the fact that he is hopelessly crippled, having lost both legs in a particularly tragic way.

In the late Middle Ages and in the Renaissance the plague was obviously a popular literary subject. Boccaccio described it most graphically in the introduction to his *Decameron* and made it the excuse for his collection of stories. The Elizabethan physician and writer William Bullein published in 1564 *A Dialogue against the Fever Pestilence* which was not only a didactic play but also showed how various people react in the proximity of death. The plague continued to haunt people's minds after it had disappeared from the West. Daniel Defoe's *Journal of the Plague Year* of 1722 was long considered an historical document, which it is not. Defoe was five years old when plague befell England for the last time. It actually is a romance, but early childhood reminiscences may have inspired the author. The romantic novelists naturally made use of such a dramatic motive as the plague, and it occurs in such gruesome stories as William Harrison Ainsworth's *Old St. Paul* of 1841. If a novelist wants to picture the plague today he must transfer the scene to China as A. J. Cronin did in *The Keys of the Kingdom,* a novel in which he packed all conceivable catastrophies between the covers of one book.

In 17th century fiction gout was a very popular subject. The disease was apparently widespread, particularly among the upper classes. Thomas Sydenham wrote a classical monograph on the subject in 1681. He was very familiar with the disease because he suffered from it himself for a long time. Gout was used in literature and in art as a characteristic of the *bon vivant* of the Falstaff type, because the popular mind attributed the disease to an abuse of wine, women, and song. Gout was popular with satirical writers and artists for another reason also. The attack of gout causes one of the most excruciating pains a man can suffer so that it certainly is anything but funny, yet it does not kill him. When the attack is over he becomes his old self again and the pain is soon forgotten. There is a contradiction between the extreme violence of the symptoms and their relative harmlessness which creates a comical situation. The same is true for the toothache, and dental patients undergoing the torture of having a tooth pulled—without anesthesia, of course—were a favorite subject of Dutch satirical painters of the 17th century. The pain caused by an attack of angina pectoris is different because such an attack kills. There the vehemence of the pain is proportionate to the danger that threatens the patient and such a situation is tragic.

Fever diseases were still extremely frequent in the 18th century. In Europe and America malaria was not limited to the southern sections but spread far to the north. Typhoid fever was endemic in every country. Fevers occur in a great many works of fiction of the period. They were the most convenient diseases to incapacitate a personage for any length of time desired and to make his condition appear just as harmless or serious as the plot required. They are usually described in very vague terms.

The romanticists, when they did not delve into the Middle Ages but treated contemporary subjects, were very fond of such languishing diseases as tuberculosis and chlorosis. The latter, an anemia of young girls, has completely disappeared today.[5] It has been attributed to the effect of the corset on the adolescent organism, but there is no doubt that other factors were involved. Chlorosis was the disease of the young girl of the upper classes who lived an indoor life without physical exercise, doing some needle work, playing some music and waiting for the husband to relieve her. It was the pale, ethereal girl, dear to the poets of the time.

Tuberculosis in those days attacked all groups of society, and many of the romantic writers suffered from it. It was usually pictured as a hereditary disease that developed slowly while the patients remained intensely interested in life—and sex. But it was the inexorable fate and therefore deeply tragic. In some novels phthisis killed rapidly—David Copperfield's young wife died of it within a few weeks—but these were exceptions. As a rule, the disease was described as chronic, destroying a human life slowly but without mercy.

In the second half of the 19th century with the advent of naturalism a new situation arose, as we shall see in a moment. At all times, however, certain diseases were in the foreground, and it is interesting to see that there is a certain relation between the prevailing diseases of a given period and their general character and style. The Middle Ages was a period of collectivism and the dominating diseases were such collective diseases as leprosy, plague, or dancing mania that befell entire groups. In the highly individualistic Renaissance syphilis was in the foreground, a disease that does not attack just anybody, but is acquired through a highly individualistic act. The Baroque period was one of tremendous contrasts and contradictions. It was the time of absolutism in France and Spain, but also of democracy in England and Holland; the time of rationalism with Descartes, but also of religious fanaticism with the Counter-Reformation. The diseases most frequently pictured were deficiency diseases such as hunger-typhus and ergotism, and luxury diseases such as gout and dropsy.

The writer of fiction who introduced a disease into his narrative was obviously influenced by his time, but then also by his purpose. If he wanted to eliminate a personage rapidly he had recourse to some acute disease such as pneumonia, or a heart disease

186

that came conveniently out of the blue sky as a stroke. If his purpose was to mark a crisis in a man's life, he pictured a serious acute disease that resulted in recovery: a brain fever, meningitis, or whatever it was meant to be, or some similar disease. A nondescript fever, headaches, or vapors were sufficient to characterize a person as sickly. Before the middle of the 19th century writers were restrained in the picturing of disease conditions. They did not describe more symptoms than were absolutely necessary to hint at the nature of a disease, omitting its unaesthetic, repulsive aspects. Things changed with the advent of naturalism.

The rise of science in the 19th century had repercussions in every cultural field. In 1865 the French physiologist Claude Bernard [6] wrote a book that was widely read by scientists and laymen alike and is still read today. It was an "Introduction to the Study of Experimental Medicine" in which the principles of the new medical science were formulated in a most persuasive way. It was a positive science, based on reason. "In one word," said Claude Bernard, "in the experimental method, just as everywhere, the only real criterion is Reason." "The mind reasons always in the same way and by the same physiological process." Reasoning, however, follows a guiding principle and this is "the absolute determinism of the phenomena." "It would be the negation of science to assume that there are facts without cause or at least without relation to other facts."

When Claude Bernard performed his experiments at the Collège de France, his audience included not only physiologists but also chemists like Marcelin Berthelot, philosophers like Paul Janet, and historians like Ernest Renan.

At about the same time, from 1861 to 1864, the French clinician Armand Trousseau published *Leçons de Clinique Médicale de l'Hôtel-Dieu* in which the principles of the new science were applied to clinical medicine. It was a strictly medical book that contained nothing but case histories, minutely described; but the two volumes found many readers outside the medical profession. A well written clinical case history is, after all, nothing but a biography. Trousseau's clinics and somewhat later those of the neurologist Charcot at the Salpêtrière were attended not only by medical students and physicians but by writers, philosophers, historians, by scientists and scholars from all fields.

Of all the sciences medicine and particularly physiology had probably the strongest appeal to the layman. Few people ever come into contact with higher mathematics or astronomy, but everybody sooner or later has some experience with medicine. The physician is the scientist whom everybody meets, and his prestige was growing rapidly in the 19th century. He demonstrated graphically to what good use the new sciences could be put. Medicine, leading through all the heights and depths of human life captivated the people's minds more than physics or chemistry. And of all medical sciences physiology was the most philosophical, for physiology investigates the functions of life, and all of its problems lead ultimately into the realm of philosophy.

The repercussions were soon felt. Renan declared history to be a science like chemistry. Hippolyte Taine, who formulated the theory and philosophy of the naturalistic school, went so far as to say that vice and virtue were products like vitriol or sugar. From Auguste Comte and Claude Bernard he derived his theory of individual determinism by environment. Auguste Comte, taking over the concept, had enlarged it to designate "not only the fluid in which the organism is dipped but at large the sum total of external circumstances of any kind, necessary for the existence of every definite organism." Claude Bernard added to this the concept of the internal environment. While the organism as a whole has an external *milieu*, every cell has an internal one that determines its development. The influence of science and particularly of medicine was most strongly felt in literature. In *La Légende des Siècles* Victor Hugo in 1859 already declared that the mission of the poet and philosopher was to try to handle social facts as the naturalist does zoological facts. Flaubert stated that according to him a novel must be scientific.

The early novels of the school were more or less clinical case histories. In *Soeur Philomène* of 1861 the brothers Goncourt pictured the life in hospital and clinic; in *Germinie Lacerteux* of 1865 the life of a woman of the lower classes. The latter novel begins characteristically with a preface-manifesto in which the authors warn the reader that this is not a faked but a true novel, that it has no happy end, that it is a study, *la clinique de l'amour*. Similarly Émile Zola's early novel *Thérèse Raquin* of 1867 was a case history describing the animal instincts of a primitive individual. In 1880 Zola wrote a treatise *Le Roman Expérimental* which he thus named in analogy to Claude Bernard's book. His thesis was that the novel must be scientific and experimental describing human beings as they are, conditioned by their environment, and analyzing the mechanism of human passions, thus constituting studies in applied sociology.

The followers of this school were not afraid of picturing the brutal and ugly aspects of life. On the contrary, they seemed to revel in doing so, feeling that this was a side of life that literature had neglected in the past. This explains why so many of them were interested in medicine, read medical books and attended clinics. Diseases occur frequently in their works and are described in a most realistic manner. When Madame Bovary in Flaubert's novel takes arsenic we are not spared any symptom. Her pulse, perspiration, spasms, and vomitings are minutely recorded. The author is not afraid to use technical language. When Homais, the pharmacist, reports to the consulting physician he says:

> Nous avons eu d'abord un sentiment de siccité au pharynx, puis des douleurs intolérables à l'épigastre, superpurgation, coma.

In the novels of Émile Zola disease, all kinds of diseases, are discussed as crudely as could be. *Lourdes* is full of nauseating details, but so is life. In *Fécondité,* a novel that glorifies maternity and the large family, the evils of abortion are branded pitilessly. *L'Assommoir* pictures the ravages of alcoholism, and the description of the attack of *delirium tremens* that kills Coupeau at the end of the book is a regular clinical case history. Zola called the twenty novels he wrote on the Rougon-Macquart family *Histoire Naturelle et Sociale d'une Famille sous le Second Empire.* He endeavored to apply scientific methods to a sociological study. The last novel of the cycle is characteristically the story of a physician *Le Docteur Pascal* who sums up the whole series and studies the heredity of the family.

I like Zola because he was a courageous fighter. He had not the detached attitude towards life that Flaubert had. He took sides passionately. Through all that mass of filth and brutality that he pictured, there is a steady outcry for a better, for a clean and healthy world built on the foundation of Fertility, Labor, Truth and Justice—the titles of his last novels.

The naturalist school had no inhibitions in regard to disease. Syphilis that had been mentioned openly in the literature of the Renaissance and Baroque had disappeared from polite literature. It came back and was brought to the stage in Ibsen's *Ghosts,* a play which describes the curse of a congenital disease, and in such plays as Eugène Brieux's *Les Avariés,* a propaganda play that pictured the effect of syphilis on marriage.

The great interest in medicine was also evidenced by the fact that the physician and particularly the medical researcher, appeared very frequently as the hero of novels and plays. François de Curel in *La Nouvelle Idole* of 1899 dramatized the conflict of a great physician who succumbed to the temptation of experimenting on his patients until a situation arose from which he could not escape except by killing himself with his own new virus.

One branch of medicine which also developed greatly during the 19th and 20th centuries, namely psychiatry, could not but influence literature, just as psychiatry itself was greatly stimulated by literature. As a matter of fact there was a constant intercourse and exchange between the two. Dostoevski was not a psychiatrist, yet he gave masterly descriptions of psychopaths, of epileptics and criminals. The fact that he was a psychopath and epileptic himself may have sharpened his senses. The same is true of the Danish writer August Strindberg whose novels are also in many ways documents of psychopathology.

The link between literature and psychiatry is easily apparent. The writer studies the life that surrounds him: people, their thoughts, emotions, passions, conflicts, and actions. All people are different; some are unusual and they and their actions attract the writer's attention particularly. There is no sharp borderline between mental health and disease, and since the overwhelming majority of neurotic individuals is not confined to institutions the writer has ample opportunity to study them. In writing he recreates them, and if he is a good writer his picture is true. In understanding and interpreting them he is, consciously or not, influenced by the psychological and psychiatric views of his day.

The psychiatrist also studies individuals, but with a different purpose in mind. He wants to cure them or at least to improve their condition. His case histories are naturally much more detailed than those of a surgeon and sometimes come very close to the character of a novel. In works of literature he occasionally finds a typical psychological situation described so perfectly that he can refer to it. The Oedipus complex is an example.

The discovery of neuroses in the 19th century and particularly the studies on hysteria carried out by Charcot and his school at the Salpêtrière in Paris and by Bernheim and his school at Nancy opened up new horizons and had far reaching repercussions. They

191

were scientific. Science was applied to study the normal and pathological functioning of the mind. We have seen that Charcot's clinic was a weekly event that attracted wide circles of Paris intellectuals. The influence on the novel was unmistakable. Paul Bourget is an exponent of the psychological trend that developed in literature in the last two decades of the 19th century. He wrote a refined style and his novels all center around the conservative catholic upper class, what the French used to call the "high-life." Nevertheless a book like *Le Disciple* published in 1889 is in its way just as brutal as any of Zola's novels. It pictures how a young psychologist seduces a girl in cold blood, systematically as an experiment, in order to apply and test his master's doctrines.

The treatment and study of hysteria was the starting point of psychoanalysis. Two Viennese physicians, Josef Breuer and Sigmund Freud, both of whom had worked with Charcot in the eighteen eighties, used, like many others, hypnosis in the treatment of hysteria. But while the classical treatment consisted in making suggestions to the hypnotic patients, they encouraged them to talk freely and found that in the hypnotic state patients were able to reproduce memories of past experiences that explained the disease condition. In thus talking spontaneously, patients discharged a considerable amount of emotions and felt relieved. Freud and Breuer called their method the "cathartic method" and published a book on the subject in 1895. It contained the discovery of the unconscious and its significance in the genesis of neuroses.

Freud abandoned hypnosis because he found other and better methods of obtaining access to the unconscious: the analysis of what patients said when they talked at random following free associations, or the interpretation of dreams. And gradually he developed his system of analyzing the mind. He was widely opposed and had enthusiastic followers, but no matter whether one accepted his system as a whole or not, nobody can deny that he has tremendously enriched psychology and psychopathology. He has opened up vast new horizons. The existence and significance of the unconscious, that enormous mass of experience hidden and forgotten—yet still acting on us—the significance of sexuality in infancy and childhood, these and so many other discoveries have become common property.

It is obvious that such a broadened psychological outlook had a considerable influence on literature. Whether writers actually studied the works of Freud or not is unimportant. Many of them directly or indirectly came under the spell of his teachings. A series of novels like Marcel Proust's *A la Recherche du Temps Perdu* is inconceivable without Freud, whose influence is strongly felt also in the works of such writers as James Joyce, Virginia Woolf, Eugene O'Neill and many others.

I am well aware that the subject of Disease and Literature is far from exhausted by these few remarks but space forbids developing it still further. I may mention only a few more points that should be considered in this connection.

In many works of fiction disease occurs incidentally in the evolution of the plot. In others, however, disease or an infirmity play a dominating part. The fact that the hero of Somerset Maugham's greatest novel, *Of Human Bondage,* has a club foot is not incidental but all important. It explains his inferiority complex and many of his actions. There is no more stirring scene than when the headmaster of his school refuses to flog him because he is a cripple. In Thomas Mann's *Magic Mountain* tuberculosis is the *leitmotif.* The novel pictures most graphically the moral and intellectual antics of the tubercular patients confined to a high altitude sanatorium.

Novels and plays were sometimes written on medical subjects in order to propagate a cause. Brieux's *Les Avariés,* mentioned before, belongs to this category. Sir Rider Haggard's *Dr. Therne* was a plea for vaccination. The *Medicine Show,* performed in New York a few years ago, was a *Living Newspaper Play* advocating the socialization of medical services. The artistic value of such works may not be very great, but they nevertheless fulfill an important function.

Medicine has been satirized, often very bitterly, at all times from the Roman poets down to G. B. Shaw. The attack was sometimes directed at the patient, as in Molière's *Le Malade Imaginaire,* but much more often at the physician. Samuel Butler's *Erewhon* of 1872, a Utopia in which criminals receive treatment and sick people are punished, was a wholesome reaction against the glorification of suffering popular with the romanticists.

At present there is, particularly in America, a vogue for novels with medical subjects. The public seems to have an unlimited capacity for absorbing them. The fashion probably started with Sinclair Lewis' *Arrowsmith.* The modern hospital and laboratory fascinate people, and there is no doubt that there is a strong dramatic element in the life and work of the men and women who in a hospital are constantly at grips with death. Some of these books are written by physicians and some by laymen. Some are good and some are very poor, following a conventional pattern. Some use the hospital merely as background for a sentimental love story, others discuss problems of medicine. In my department at the Johns Hopkins University we buy all these books although we rarely read them. We feel, however, that some day they will make interesting documents. And this raises the question whether works of fiction may be used as sources of medical history.

The answer is yes, if such books are consulted critically and used with discrimination. Homer did not intend to write a treatise on medicine, but his epics obviously mention wounds, diseases and their treatment and thus reflect medical views of the time. As long as medicine was not a specialized science but the common property of the educated classes, ideas expressed on medical subjects by poets must be considered carefully. The Greek tragic poets thus are an important source of medical history.

In reading satirical writers one must remember that they always exaggerate. The physicians of Molière's days were not as bad as he pictured them. Yet the account he gives of them is true, and the satire was perfectly justified. A new science was developing in the 17th century, while the universities retained their mediaeval character. The average physician behaved and reasoned like a doctor of the Middle Ages and was unaware of the new science. This produced a comical situation that Molière exploited adding to it his personal grudges against the profession.[7]

Memoirs, diaries, letters and similar documents are very revealing sources. The diaries of Pepys, the letters of Madame de Sévigné, for instance, are full of accounts of diseases and their treatments. They give us a picture of medicine seen from the patient's angle.

NOTES

1. See Benedetto Croce, *Theory and History of Historiography*, London, 1921.

2. Lewis J. Moorman, *Tuberculosis and Genius*, Chicago, 1940.

3. Dr. Herbert Silvette, of the University of Virginia, is preparing a bibliography of works dealing with medicine in English literature which will be found extremely useful.

4. See e. g. George M. Gould, *Biographic Clinics*, 6 vols., Philadelphia, 1903–1909.

5. Axel Hansen, *Om Chlorosens, den aegte Blegsots, Optraeden i Europa*, Kolding, 1928.

6. About him see the excellent book of J. M. D. Olmsted, *Claude Bernard Physiologist*, New York, 1938.

7. See O. Temkin, Studien zum "Sinn"-Begriff in der Medizin, *Kyklos*, 1929, Vol. II, p. 66 ff.

CHAPTER X

Disease and Art

DISEASE is a dynamic process. It has a beginning—slow or sudden—develops, reaches in many cases an acme, and ends in recovery or death. Disease, therefore, can be described in words. It is a highly epical and sometimes dramatic subject, but the artist who tries to picture disease in a painting or sculpture is greatly handicapped by the fact that he can reproduce only one moment of the process.

The cinema which combines art and literature, could portray disease in time. Some interesting experiments have been made along that line as, for instance, the Swiss film *The Eternal Mask*. As long, however, as the movies consider themselves an industry with the sole purpose of providing cheap entertainment, we cannot expect much. Yet I could think of unusually interesting subjects, such as the fever phantasies of a man stricken with disease at a crucial moment of his life. The hallucinations of a patient suffering from *delirium tremens* would provide more horrors than any murder story and would be good propaganda against alcoholism.

When does an artist picture disease and why? [1] One reason for doing it was at all times the demand for portraits. People wished to have their likeness reproduced for relatives and friends—and for posterity. The artist, of course, did not make the portrait of an individual while he was suffering from an acute disease, but if his subject happened to be afflicted with a chronic disease or in-

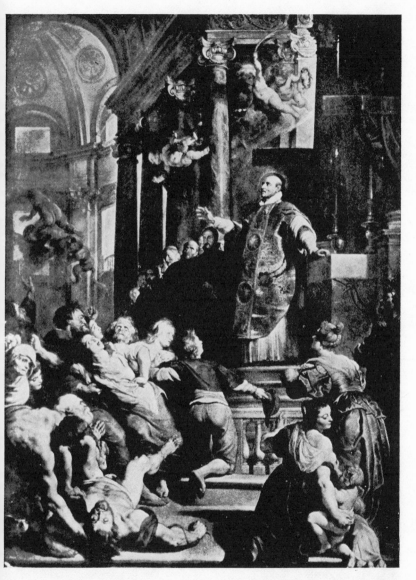

35. ST. IGNATIUS CURING THE POSSESSED AND REVIVING
THE CHILDREN. (Painting by Rubens, at the Vienna Museum.)

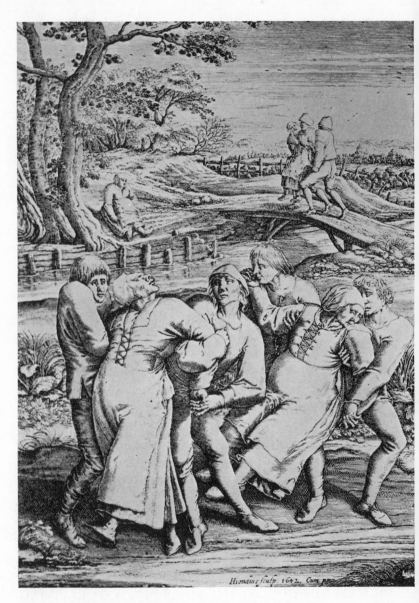

36. ST. VITUS DANCERS. (After a painting by Peter Breughel the Elder.)

firmity, the artist had no choice. He was forced to picture the person in his diseased condition. Thus we possess a large number of portraits representing a great variety of ailments. The Egyptian Chnoum-hotep who around 2700 B. C. was in charge of the Royal Wardrobe, was a dwarf and his portrait statuette in the Museum of Cairo shows unmistakably that his condition was the result of *achondroplasia,* a disturbance in the development of the cartilage. The funeral stele of the priest Ruma who lived at the time of the 18th dynasty shows a highly atrophied right leg. Such atrophies frequently occur in the course of poliomyelitis but may also be due to other diseases of the nervous system. One has to be very cautious in diagnosing a disease from a work of art. The artist may have pictured his subject very realistically, yet unless the visible symptoms are quite characteristic, it is impossible to make more than a tentative diagnosis. A diagnosis is highly desirable, however, particularly in the case of early historical works of art of a period when literary medical documents are scanty. A picture or statue may then be the only evidence of the incidence of a certain disease. Thus we have no descriptions of tuberculosis from ancient Egypt but we know with certainty that the disease occurred. We have a funeral statuette representing a highly emaciated man with a hunchback who in all probability suffered from Pott's disease, a form of tuberculosis.[2] But in that case we have more: we have several Egyptian mummies showing the same condition,[3] and the microscopic examination of one of them even revealed traces of an abscess along the spinal column which makes the diagnosis certain.

The portrait painter, of course, does not emphasize his model's infirmities, but when they affect the face, he cannot avoid them. Lucas of Leyden in painting Ferdinand of Spain, gave a splendid illustration of what adenoids do to a man's looks. Affections of the nose such as rhinophyma and rhinoscleroma have been represented very graphically by various Dutch painters of the 17th century. The realism in a portrait may be such that even internal diseases which do not alter the outlines of the body may become evident. An anecdote relates that the great clinician Corvisart, Napoleon's body physician, once said in looking at a portrait: "If this picture is a faithful one, I cannot doubt that the original must have died of heart disease," which had actually happened.

The Biblical tradition and the traditions of the Church provided artists with a great variety of pathological subjects. Christ curing the sick was represented endless times, and this gave the artist an opportunity to picture the blind, the lame, the leper, the demoniac, all the sick who had approached Christ in the hope of being healed. But not only Jesus—his apostles and all the saints had also performed miraculous cures. As long as religion was the chief source of inspiration to the artist and provided the great majority of his motives, the treatment of sick people was a very popular subject, and the artist pictured them the way he saw them in his immediate environment.

Since many saints were patrons protecting man against specific diseases, they appear with special attributes or in the act of curing patients afflicted with that special disease. St. Roch is usually pointing at the plague bubo that had developed in his groin. St. Lazarus is pictured as a leper. St. Elizabeth, who devoted her life to the nursing of the sick, appears in many paintings and sculptures while she is attending to lepers. Such pictures inspired the people who prayed to the saint for intervention and confirmed them in their faith. The Middle Ages glorified poverty and illness, looked upon them as meritorious conditions helping the people toward salvation. Care of the sick and poor was extolled, and as a result of this attitude mediaeval works of art abound with representations of beggars, cripples and the sick in both mind and body.

The healing of demoniacs by Christ or a saint was a favorite subject of mediaeval artists and for long thereafter. It was a particularly spectacular cure, that of a man raving with madness from whom the evil spirit escaped all of a sudden. Mental patients who became violent were kept in bonds, and the artists in order to indicate their madness usually represented them handcuffed, chained or held by several persons. The cure was effected by touching the patient or, more often, by exorcising the evil spirit. In such a case the saint was pictured holding his hand over the victim while he pronounced the magic words. More primitive methods were also applied: thus on a 14th century fresco in San Miniato, St. Benedict is flogging a possessed monk in order to drive out the spirit.

The result of the cure was indicated in the Middle Ages by picturing the demon as he escaped through the mouth of the victim, or sometimes through the head. The earliest pictures preserved, dating from the 5th and 6th centuries, show the demon in the shape of a small, winged human being, as the Greeks had represented the soul, or sometimes as a bird. Later, when the devil had assumed the features of the Greek Pan, the demons became more picturesque with hoofs, horns, a tail and the wings of a bat. In the Renaissance the devil may still appear on the picture but not at the moment when he is leaving the victim's body, as this would spoil the design. He instead appears flying through the air or in a corner of the picture on his way back to hell. Usually, however, the crucial moment of the cure is indicated by the violent contortions of the victim.

The drama of such scenes greatly appealed to the painters of the Baroque period. Rubens, who had been a student of the Jesuits in Antwerp, left two large paintings and several sketches representing St. Ignatius of Loyola exorcising demoniacs and at the same time resuscitating dead children. The pictures, particularly the one in Vienna, are extremely dramatic, contrasting the quiet felicity of the mothers whose children came back to life with the horribly contorted bodies of the possessed. Similarly, on a painting of Jordaens in the Museum of Brussels representing St. Martin healing a demoniac, the serenity of the saint, the tense curiosity of the Roman proconsul who was to be converted by this miracle, and the convulsions of the possessed who can barely be held by four strong persons, form a highly theatrical contrast.

Peter Breughel's sketches of dancing maniacs are of a somewhat different order. The dancing mania or St. Vitus' dance apparently was a mass hysteria that swept in repeated epidemics particularly through the Rhinelands in the 14th and 15th centuries.[4] Hundreds of people, men and women, suddenly seized by this strange craze, would start out on pilgrimages to the chapel of St. Vitus in Zabern or to St. Willibrod in Echternach dancing steadily to the music of bagpipes. They were considered possessed and were exorcised, but the mania flared up repeatedly even after the 15th century, and the memory of it was perpetuated in a procession held annually at Echternach on the Tuesday following Whitsuntide. Breughel must have witnessed such an event. He pictured the victims, marching in dance steps, in groups of three, a woman in the middle flanked by two men, looking as if they were intoxicated.

We mentioned in a previous chapter that the saints were not the only miraculous healers, and that the kings of France and England performed such cures also, particularly on those suffering from scrofula. It is obvious that the artists did not miss a subject that was so flattering to royalty, and the only reason why more paintings were not devoted to such scenes is that the custom was limited to two courts. There are pictures on the subject, however, such as the painting of Bernaert van Orley representing the anointment of a French king, while in the courtyard outside the sick are waiting to be touched. Since the painter, however, had not

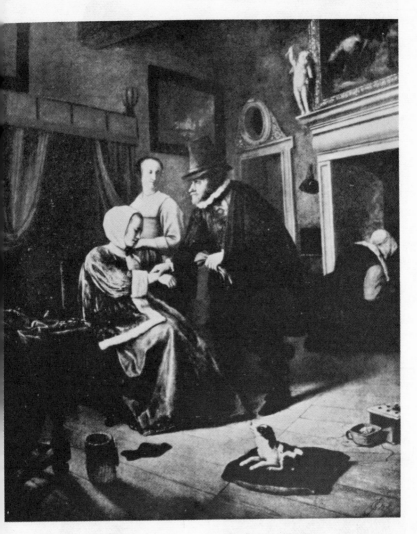

37. PHYSICIAN AND PATIENT. (Painting by Jan Steen. Museum in The Hague.)

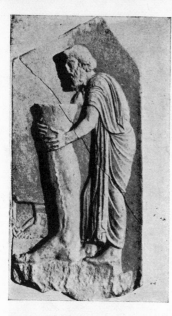

38. VARICOSE LEG. (Votive relief from the Asclepius temple in Athens.)

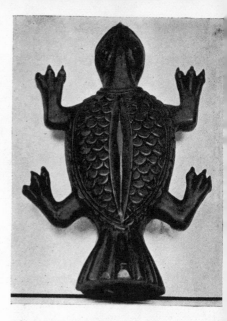

39. WAX TOAD REPRESENTING THE UTERUS. (Ex-voto from Bavaria.)

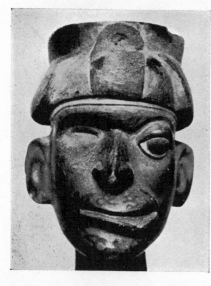

40. PERUVIAN HUACO REPRESENTING A FACIAL PARALY-

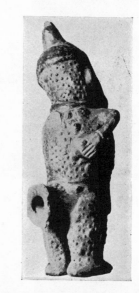

41. PERUVIAN HUACO REPRESENTING A SKIN DISEASE

much experience with scrofula, he pictured the patients with the features of lepers.

The story of Tobias also appears frequently in pictures. Once he went to sleep near the wall under a swallows' nest and hot excrements of the birds fell into his eyes. Thus God made him blind in order to try him like Job. But the angel Raphael revealed to young Tobias, the son, that bile of a fish would restore his father's eyesight.

> "Then Tobias took fish bile and applied it to his father's eyes. He kept it for almost half an hour; then a white matter began to come out from his eyes like the skin of an egg. When Tobias saw it, he drew it from his father's eyes, who immediately recovered his eyesight." [5]

An etching of Rembrandt represents the scene that preceded the cure. The blind father hearing his son approach hurries to welcome him, but being blind, he misses the door. Most pictures, however, illustrate the treatment, young Tobias rubbing fish bile into the old man's eyes, or removing the skin from his eyes, in very much the same way as an oculist would remove a cataract.

And finally I would like to mention in this connection that in illustrating Biblical scenes artists also pictured women in childbirth and in childbed. The birth of Jesus being a miraculous one was, of course, out of the question, but Anna giving birth to Mary was a very popular subject. These paintings give us a very good idea of what a delivery room looked like in various periods. They show us the posture of the parturient, the midwives at work, the bath being prepared for the child and an infinity of little details that are usually rarely mentioned in books because they were taken for granted.[6]

The desire to illustrate the Biblical and the clerical traditions was for a very long time the chief motive for the representation of sick people in art, but disease conditions were also pictured independently and for various reasons. Such a curse as leprosy, a catastrophe like an epidemic of plague, could not but stir the imagination of artists.

It is not by accident that we have to mention these two diseases in almost every chapter of this book. Their grip on mankind for centuries was such that they affected every aspect of civilization. The signs of leprosy were visible. The disease affected the skin, mutilated the face and the extremities, and people lived with these signs branded on them for decades, rotting away slowly. The horror of such a condition attracted artists who wanted to paint the dark sides of life. But it was still more the inexorability of the leper's fate, the deep tragedy of his life, that made him the subject of so many paintings. In the *Triumph of Death* once attributed to Orcagna, in the Campo Santo of Pisa, Death, an ugly winged figure, passes by a group of poor lepers and reaches out for another group, young men and women in the prime of life who sing and play music, unaware of the proximity of death. In vain the lepers are calling for it to relieve them, stretching out their arms, mutilated with claw hands. Death has no regard for them, and their misery will continue for years to come.

Less dramatic but still more tragic is a painting by Nicolaus Manuel Deutsch in the Museum of Basle. In the foreground is a beautiful young woman richly dressed. She seems in perfect health, yet on her left forearm is a nodule, a leproma, the beginning of the disease. Behind her stands a man in rags with emaciated body, the legs elephantiastically swollen, the arms mutilated, the face disfigured so as to give him the typical leonine expression—the beginning and end of the disease. We see what fate has in store for the young woman and we shudder.

The plague-ridden sick were not good subjects for the artist; people suffering from acute diseases never are. The sick room of so highly contagious a patient was avoided whenever possible. We have seen that St. Roch was usually pictured with a plague bubo in the groin, but this had the value of a symbol and was a mere attribute. The saint otherwise does not appear as a man prostrated by a deadly disease. There are pictures of the plague by Raphael and particularly by Baroque artists. As a rule they represent mass scenes, with people dying in the streets and others fleeing terror-stricken. It is the social and psychological aspect of the disease that appears on such paintings rather than its physical symptoms.

The influence of the plague on art manifested itself much more strongly in a totally different way. It was a great stimulation. An epidemic of plague in a community was a stirring collective experience. At such a time people made vows, to be fulfilled when the plague was over by erecting altars to St. Sebastian and St. Roch, or by building votive churches like Santa Maria della Salute in Venice. Many Baroque churches were built all over Europe as a result of such vows. In Austria the plague gave rise to a special kind of monument, the plague columns, *Pestsäulen*. The best known is that in Vienna, dedicated to the Holy Trinity. It was built of Salzburg marble, in the years 1687–1693, by Fischer von Erlach, following sketches of the architect and theatrical engineer Burnacini, in fulfillment of a vow made during the plague of 1679. The same type of columns can be found in Baden, Heiligenkreuz and a number of other Austrian towns. They are among the most striking expressions of the South German Baroque.

While leprosy and plague were two major subjects, there were other abnormal conditions of the human body that attracted the artists. Velasquez and other painters of the Spanish school never wearied of picturing all conceivable varieties of idiots, and they did it so realistically that in most cases it is possible to diagnose the kind of idiocy represented. The Dutch painters of the 17th century reveled in reproducing everyday life with all its joys and miseries. Their pictures are full of good and rich food, strong drinks, dances, merriment and fist fights. Ailments of heart and body are represented also—never too seriously. In the paintings by Jan Steen, Gabriel Metsu, van Hoogstraaten, van Mieris, Gerard Dou and many others the patient is usually a young woman, pale and languid. The physician seems to delight in feeling her pulse or in examining the urine. You are never quite sure whether the woman's trouble is caused by a disease such as chlorosis or melancholia, or by the very tangible results of love. There is a satirical touch in many of these pictures, and still more so in paintings such as that of Adriaen Brouwer, picturing a man making horrible faces after tasting a bitter remedy, or in the many scenes where a poor devil's aching tooth is being pulled. There is a straight line of development from these pictures to the bitter satires of Hogarth and Rowlandson. Medicine always had its shortcomings and failures. In every man's life there comes the final disease against which there is *nulla herba in ortis*. At all times greedy physicians exploited the sufferings of their patients, and satirical artists hammered at them as they did at the shyster lawyer and other professions. On such pictures patients are represented, fat ones and lean ones, those suffering from dropsy, and gout and other diseases. The attack, however, is not directed at them but at their doctors.

When a patient had been cured by Asclepius, he frequently expressed his gratitude by presenting the temple with a votive offering. People of means sometimes had large reliefs made in marble by artists of renown. They represented the god, alone or in the company of one of his children Hygeia or Telesphorus; and in front of him in much smaller size was the suppliant with family members and servants carrying gifts. Sometimes the healing act was pictured. A votive relief from the Asklepieion of Athens shows the patient sleeping on a couch, his head on pillows. The god stands nearby leaning on his staff and one of his servants is operating on the patient's head. This in all probability was a true picture of the dream that the sick man had had.

Patients of more moderate means could not afford such lavish gifts. They gave a modest sculpture representing the part of the body that had been ailing them, the head, the eyes, the breasts, the intestines, the extremities or some other part. They were crudely made according to the popular anatomical views of the day, were produced wholesale, and could be bought in shops in the vicinity of the temples. Sometimes these votives were made of gold or silver, and the temples kept inventories of these more precious gifts. An inscription from the Asclepius temple of Athens mentions over one hundred such votive offerings representing eyes alone. Most votives made from precious metals have disappeared for obvious reasons, but thousands made from marble or terra cotta have been preserved and can be seen in every museum that has Graeco-Roman collections. They have been found all over the ancient world, not only in temples of Asclepius but of other deities. Many have been found in Italy in Etruscan excavations.

Of particular interest to us in this chapter is the fact that many such votive offerings represent not the normal but the diseased organ. Some are very crude and merely indicate vaguely a tumor or an ulcer, but others are quite elaborate and must have been specially made for an individual patient. A votive relief from the Asklepieion of Athens shows a man, obviously the patient, holding a large leg with a varicose vein. Skin eruptions, deformities of the fingers and other pathological conditions have been represented on votive offerings in a similar way.

The custom of presenting temples with such offerings survived the downfall of ancient civilization and was taken over by the Church. Just as the pagan had done in the past, the Christian went to the Church, prayed and sacrificed for healing and donated a votive offering when he felt restored. They can be seen in many churches even today. The cheap ones are made of wax, representing heart, lungs, eyes, or legs. In the Alpine countries the toad symbolized the uterus, and white or red wax toads frequently appear there among the votives, donated by women who had been relieved from gynecological troubles or who had become pregnant after a long period of sterility. Among these votives, embroideries or paintings are also often found, representing a sick man in bed or an accident that would have been fatal without the intervention of the saint. They are naive expressions of popular art.

Popular handicraft was also responsible for an extraordinarily rich material that has come down to us from ancient Peru, the *huacos*. Huacos are pottery drinking vessels that were used by the Incas. Like the Egyptians, the Incas provided their dead with all the utensils that they might have needed in the hereafter. Among them were many examples of such earthenware, and hundreds of them have been excavated in ancient burial grounds and can be seen in museums today. These huacos represent all aspects of life. Some have the shape of heads of great beauty, others of entire figures. Some reproduce erotic scenes, or the birth of a child, and many of them represent a great variety of disease conditions very realistically, as if the artists had had a morbid interest in abnormalities. Among the collections of the Berlin Museum of Ethnology that I once studied is a huaco with the head of a man suffering from facial paralysis, another that shows a rash extending over the whole body while the patient is scratching himself. Many others picture deep ulcers of the face reminiscent of lupus or possibly of syphilis. Blind men, invalids, and death masks appear in the form of such pottery, a gruesome collection which, however, reveals a keen sense of observation.

A word should be said about medical illustration, which is also art and always reflects the style of its period. The rise of anatomy would have been impossible without the cooperation of artists.

Leonardo da Vinci's anatomical drawings come to mind at once but he was not alone. The many illustrators known and unknown have in all probability contributed infinitely more to medical science than we commonly assume. A period like the Renaissance was not an age of specialism. The structure of the human body appeared as a new field that had to be conquered. The medical man had more book knowledge than the artist, to be sure, but what mattered then was what Leonardo called *saper vedere,* and the artist sometimes may have seen more than the physicians did. Vesalius is inconceivable without his artist, van Kalkar. Their names will always be linked together, and even in later centuries we hear over and over again how dependent the medical scientist was on his artists, from Haller and his illustrators to Howard Kelly and Max Broedel who at the Johns Hopkins University founded a flourishing school which for half a century supplied the United States with medical illustrators.

Anatomy, more than any other field of medical science, was in need of illustrations because anatomical structures can be described much more clearly in a drawing than in words. However, the desire to illustrate other medical conditions also was felt very early. In the first century B. C. already the commentary of Apollonius of Citium to the Hippocratic treatise on articulations was illustrated with pictures showing the various methods of reducing the dislocated joints. In the same century herbals were illustrated. As long as there was no uniform botanical nomenclature and plants were designated by an infinity of different names in every country and region, pictures were a great help in identifying them. In the 2nd century A. D. the Greek physician Soranus wrote a treatise on surgical dressings and bandages which was also accompanied by illustrations that greatly contributed to a clearer understanding of the text.

In the Middle Ages surgical books were frequently illustrated. It was much easier to show in a picture where the cautery should be applied or where venesection should be performed than in a text. With the development of pathological anatomy from the 17th century on, the demand for pictures became as imperative as it had been in normal anatomy.[7] When physicians began to differentiate more and more skin diseases, they could not possibly do without the artist. It is extremely difficult to describe a rash unequivocally in words, while a colored picture will immediately show what is meant. Many of the new diagnostic methods could not have been developed without the cooperation of artists. What the doctor's eye saw through the ophthalmoscope, uroscope, gastroscope, and similar instruments had to be pictured in atlases for didactic purposes. And the X-ray examination was entirely pictorial.

Today the photographer has, in most cases, replaced the artist, and the development of color photography permits the making of very realistic pictures. Motion picture films play an increasingly important part in medical education. Operations on small objects such as the eye can be demonstrated much better in a color film than in the operating room.

The application of photography to medical illustration undoubtedly had great advantages because the photographic lens does not lie, but it had also disadvantages. It is not always possible to direct the light in such a way that essentials will be accentuated while non-essentials will recede to the background. The photograph, while it is always true to nature, sometimes has too many details and thus may be confusing. Hence there is still a definite need for medical illustrators, particularly for publications of a didactic character.

In 1921 the German psychiatrist Hans Prinzhorn published an extremely interesting book which he called *Bildnerei der Geisteskranken, ein Beitrag zur Psychologie und Psychopathologie der Gestaltung*.[8] He was working at the Psychiatric Clinic in Heidelberg and examined thousands of drawings, paintings, and sculp-

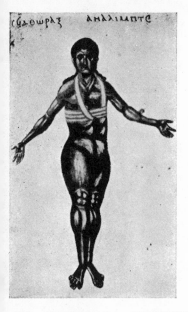

42. SURGICAL DRESSING. (From Soranus, Florence MS. Laurent. LXXIV 7, 9th–10th century.)

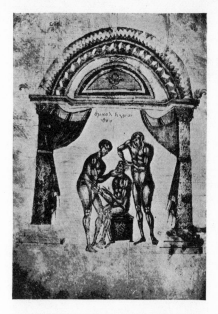

43. REDUCTION OF THE DISLOCATED JAW. (From Apollonius of Kitium, Florence MS. Laurent. LXXIV 7, 9th–10th century.)

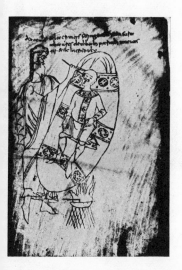

44. MEDIAEVAL CAUTERIZATION. (Florence MS. LXXIII 41,

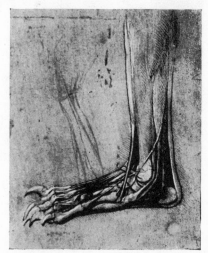

45. ANATOMICAL DRAWING BY LEONARDO DA VINCI.

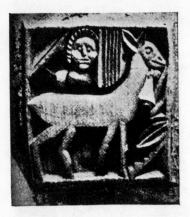

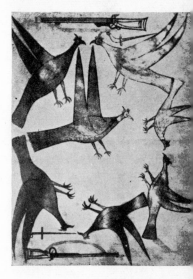

46. RELIEF BY A MENTAL PA-
TIENT.

47. DRAWING BY A MENTAL PA-
TIENT.

(From Prinzhorn, *Bildnerei der Geisteskranken*, 2. Auflage, Berlin, 1923.)

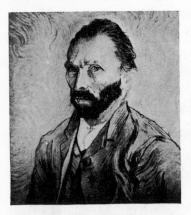

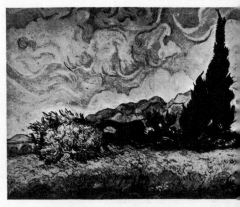

48. VINCENT VAN GOGH,
SELF PORTRAIT.

49. LANDSCAPE WITH CYPRESSES
BY VAN GOGH. (Tate Gallery, London.

tures made by mental patients, particularly patients suffering from schizophrenia.

Everybody has the urge to express himself. We do it by working, talking, writing, dancing, or performing other actions, but we can also take a pencil and draw lines and curves that seem perfectly devoid of any meaning. Actually, however, they are not meaningless but reflect a mental process, and the analysis of such drawings gives a clue to the understanding of an individual's mind just as the analysis of other expressions does. In drawing at random an individual may reveal unconscious drives, just as he does in talking at random or in dreaming.

The examination of pictures and sculptures made by schizophrenic patients showed that persons who had never received any training in art created in their psychoses works of artistic value. Still more interesting was the observation that many such pictures were similar in style and concept to those of definite historical periods. Past experiences and reminiscences of the individual may explain this phenomenon in some cases. In others, however, it is highly probable that in his psychosis the mental processes of a patient had reverted to a more primitive type and that his artistic expressions therefore revealed a more primitive style. Similar observations have been made with the drawings of children. The examination of such pictures is important medically in that it greatly helps us to understand a patient's mind, and psychoanalysis is making extensive use of this method.[9] But it is also important because it throws light on the mechanism of the creative, artistic process.

Disease never makes an artist where there is none. It may remove inhibitions, change the sense of values, and liberate forces previously hidden. When an artist suffers from a psychosis, the disease obviously reflects itself in his creations. Van Gogh is the classical example. There is some controversy as to the character of his illness. He was not only addicted to alcohol but suffered also from violent hallucination attacks followed by amnesia. In one such attack he cut off one of his ears; in another he committed suicide. Even if we had no records of his life, his self-portrait would be sufficient evidence of his disturbed mental condition. French psychiatrists usually agree that he suffered from a form of epilepsy without the typical epileptic fits. Jaspers thought of schizophrenia, Kleist and others of what they called *Episodische Dämmerzustände*.[10] When we study the development of his work from the early period to the *Black Birds* we can trace step by step the development of his genius—and of his disease.

Chronic physical diseases may also influence an artist's creations. It has been said that El Greco suffered from astigmatism and that this explained the distortions of his figures. In other words, he would have seen nature and his works with eyes that were organically different from our normal eyes.

Illness may have influenced the choice of subjects made by some artists. The painter Watteau was tubercular all his life. The many elegant ladies playing light-heartedly, the Italian comedians, the martial soldiers he painted may have been the expression of a man's pining for a life from which he was inexorably excluded, the outburst of a sick man who knew that his life was doomed.

A serious illness always profoundly affects a man's life. The proximity of death is deeply stirring, and the artist who is more sensitive than other people and whose function it is to express what he feels, cannot but react very strongly to such experiences.

NOTES

1. The relations between medicine and art have been studied very extensively by Charcot and his co-workers, particularly Paul Richer. In 1888 they launched a serial publication devoted to the subject, *Nouvelle Iconographie de la Salpêtrière*. An index of the first 18 volumes was published in 1903, *L'Oeuvre Médico-*

artistique de la Nouvelle Iconographie de la Salpêtrière. A number of valuable monographs came from the same school, such as Charcot and Paul Richer, *Les Démoniaques dans l'Art,* Paris, 1887; Charcot and Paul Richer, *Les Difformes et les Malades dans l'Art,* Paris, 1889; Paul Richer, *L'Art et la Médecine,* Paris, n.d. [1902] In Germany these studies were cultivated particularly by Eugen Holländer, *Die Medizin in der klassischen Malerei,* Stuttgart, 1903; *Die Karikatur und Satire in der Medizin,* Stuttgart, 1905; *Plastik und Medizin,* Stuttgart, 1912. See also H. E. Sigerist, The Historical Aspect of Art and Medicine, *Bulletin of the Institute of the History of Medicine,* 1936, Vol. IV, pp. 271–296.

2. Schrumpf-Pierron, Le mal de Pott en Egypte 4000 ans avant notre ère, *Aesculape,* 1933, Vol. 23, pp. 295–299.

3. Marc Armand Ruffer, *Studies in the Palaeopathology of Egypt,* Chicago, 1921, pp. 3–10.

4. Hellmuth Liebscher, *Ein Kartographischer Beitrag zur Geschichte der Tanzwut,* Leipzig Thesis, 1931.

5. Liber Tobiae, XI, 13–15.

6. See Robert Müllerheim, *Die Wochenstube in der Kunst,* Stuttgart, 1904.

7. Edgar Goldschmid, *Entwicklung und Bibliographie der pathologisch-anatomischen Abbildung,* Leipzig, 1925.

8. Berlin 1921; 2nd ed., 1923.

9. See M. G. Baynes, *Mythology of the Soul, a Research into the Unconscious from Schizophrenic Dreams and Drawings,* Baltimore, 1940.

10. V. Doiteau and E. Leroy, *La Folie de Vincent van Gogh,* Paris, 1928.—K. Jaspers, *Strindberg und van Gogh,* Berlin, 1926.—W. Riese, Vincent van Gogh in der Krankheit, *Grenzfragen des Nerven- und Seelenlebens,* Heft 125, Munich, 1926.

CHAPTER XI

Disease and Music

DISEASE and music seem to have very little in common; yet even a very cursory glance at history shows that they have always been intimately related. Some people are good musicians, others are not; but no one remains totally unaffected by music. Not everybody can appreciate the late string quartets of Beethoven or the songs of Debussy, but there are few who do not feel something when they hear a military march played by a brass band, or the joyful tunes of a Viennese waltz, or hot jazz, or the tomtom in the jungle. To many of us music is a source of profound emotion and deep happiness.

If music affects people who are in good health, it must make a still stronger impression upon the sick whose emotional balance is less stable and who are more receptive to stimulations from outside. "And it came to pass, when the evil spirit from God was upon Saul, that David took an harp, and played with his hand: so Saul was refreshed, and was well, and the evil spirit departed from him." [1] Asclepius treated sick people with drugs, with the knife and with soothing songs. Incantations were not only a sequence of magic words; they had a tune also and had to be chanted over the sick, as the word *incantatio* indicates.

Throughout antiquity music was applied in the treatment of diseases. [2] We mentioned in a previous chapter the important place that music took in the School of Pythagoras. It was used also by physicians of the Sicilian school, according to the testimony of Caelius Aurelianus: [3] "Others have approved of the use of songs (cantilenae), as the brother of Philistion also remarks in book XXII *On Remedies,* where he writes that a certain piper had played his melodies over aching parts of the body which, quivering and throbbing, were relaxed after the pain had been destroyed." The philosophers also mentioned the therapeutic use of music. There is an important passage relative to the subject in the *Attic Nights* of Aulus Gellius where he says: [4] "I ran across the statement very recently in the book of Theophrastus *On Inspiration* that many men have believed and put their belief on record, that when gouty pains in the hips are most severe they are relieved if a flute-player plays soothing measures. That snake-bites are cured by the music of the flute, when played skillfully and melodiously, is also stated in a book of Democritus entitled *On Deadly Infections,* in which he shows that the music of the flute is medicine for many ills that flesh is heir to. So very close is the connection between the bodies and the minds of men, and therefore between physical and mental ailments and their remedies." To some of these writers music appeared as a kind of psychotherapy that acted on the body through the medium of the mind. Later physicians were more skeptical, such as Soranus in the 2nd century A. D. who thought that "those people were stupid who believed that the violence of the disease could be driven out by melodies and a song (modulis et cantilena)." [5] There can be no doubt, however, that musical therapy continued to be applied, if not by physicians then by the innumerable quacks, priests and magicians who found plenty of customers in ancient Rome and also outside of the capital.

It is obvious that the custom was continued in the Middle Ages when music played such an important part in the cult, and religious medicine was so much in the foreground. The famous hymn to the Nativity of St. John the Baptist [6] attributed to Petrus Diaconus was believed to have a healing effect on colds, probably on account of its text: [7]

> Ut queant laxis resonare fibris
> Mira gestorum famuli tuorum
> Solve polluti labii reatum
> Sancte Joannes.

When people of high standing were sick, their court musicians wrote special compositions, if not to cure them, then at least to cheer them up. Once it happened that Pope Boniface VIII had to take a purgative and was to be phlebotomized. His learned court musician and poet, Bonaiutus de Casentino, commemorated the event by writing two compositions. He sent them to the Pope's physician-in-ordinary Magister Accursinus with a letter in which he asked him to show them to the Holy Father, "for I believe that he will praise the writer's devotion or—what is more likely to happen—will laugh at his fancy." The compositions are preserved in a manuscript of the Vatican from which they have been published recently.[8] The first, a kind of a ballad, has a long text in which medical and spiritual matters are intermingled freely: [9]

> Sic laventur intestina
> Quid se purget et sentina
> Mentis omni crimine.
> Tunc est digna cura cutis,
> Quando munus fert salutis
> In utroque homine.
> Cum servatur sensitiva
> Virtus et intellectiva
> Viget spes solatii.

The second is a hymn on the Pope's venaesection beginning: [10]

> Sanguis demptus et redemptus
> Nos servet in letitia.
> Qua optetur et prestetur
> Eterna celi gloria.

Pope Boniface VIII was not necessarily sick because in the

Middle Ages people used to take purgatives and were bled periodically, particularly in the spring, as a measure of hygiene. The
case was different with the Marchese Francesco Gonzaga of Man-
tua, who was the husband of Isabella d'Este, and whose court was
one of the most brilliant of the Italian Renaissance. But the Marchese was a very sick man. He suffered for many years from
syphilis, which the Italians at that time called the *morbo gallico*,
the French disease, while the French retaliated by calling it the
disease of Naples. Francesco Gonzaga died in 1519, but two
years before, in 1517, his musician and friend Marchetto Cara
composed a *frottola* for four voices on his master's illness.[11] The
frottola, like the *toscanella*, the *moresco* or the *vilanella* was a type
of song very popular in Renaissance Italy. It was derived from folk
music, and Marchetto Cara's piece, in spite of its gruesome subject
had a very simple and charming melody that must have greatly
pleased the marquis. The text begins: [12]

> Quis furor tanti rabiesque morbi
> Quae lues, quae vis animum fatigat
> Quod malum serpit, vorat ad medullas
> Dulce venenum

Music was, of course, also used in the cult of the saints who protected mankind against illness. I once found in a junk store an interesting book with music by an anonymous composer written in
praise of St. Sebastian. It had the cumbersome title:

> Vita et gesta gloriosissimi martyris Sancti Sebastiani, singularis
> contra pestem patroni. Iconibus et elogiis latino-germanicis illus-
> trata. Das ist: Leben und Thaten des Heiligen und Glorwürdigen
> Martyrers Sebastiani, sonderbahren Patronen wider die Pest. In
> Kupffer-Stichen mit Latein- und Teutschen Lob-Sprüchen öffen-
> tlich vorgestellet. Denen am End nach der ordentlichen Zahl der
> Kupffer die Musicalischen Arien mit ihren Partituren beygesetzt
> seynd. Superiorum permissu. Augspurg, zu finden bey Wilhelm
> Panegger, Buchbindern, 1702.

The text contains the Sebastian legend from his birth to his martyrdom in Latin and German verse. The music shows Italian influence. I once had it performed at the Johns Hopkins Institute of the History of Medicine.

What I particularly wish to discuss in this chapter is the history of a strange disease for which the only cure was music, namely *tarantism.*

This malady occurred in Apulia where it seems to have been localized for centuries. It was frequently mentioned in medical literature, but mostly by people who knew it only from hearsay. We are fortunate, however, in having reports from two reliable physicians who lived in Apulia, saw cases with their own eyes, and wrote detailed descriptions with case histories. One of them, Epiphanius Ferdinandus, practised medicine in Apulia for over twenty years before he published a collection of medical observations.[13] The other was Giorgio Baglivi, the leading iatromechanist of the 17th century. Born in Ragusa, he was adopted by an Apulian physician and spent part of his life in that region. At the request of the Swiss physician J. J. Manget, he wrote a short report on tarantism for the *Bibliotheca Medico-Practica,* but finding it unsatisfactory he wrote a dissertation on the subject in 1695.[14] Like Ferdinandus' book, it contains a number of very interesting case histories.

A third and important source to the subject is the work of the learned Jesuit father Athanasius Kircher *Magnes sive de Arte Magnetica Opus Tripartitum,* first published in Rome in 1641.[15] In this book dealing with all forms of magnetism one section is devoted to *The Powerful Magnetism of Music* (De Potenti Musicae Magnetismo) in which by far the longest chapter is *On Tarantism or the Apulian Spider Tarantula, its Magnetism and Strange Sympathy with Music.* Kircher had gathered information on the subject from all sources available and particularly from the personal reports sent to him by two Apulian clerics, Pater Nicolellus and Pater Gallibertus, who were both very familiar with the disease. The chief significance of Kircher's book lies in the fact that he collected the music played in the treatment of tarantism and published it so that it has come down to us.

Although individual cases of the disease seem to have occurred in other sections of Italy and in Spain, it was otherwise localized in Apulia, a very hot region in the heel of the Italian boot. Baglivi describes it in the following words: "The above-mentioned Apulia lies eastward and stands exposed to the eastern and northerly winds. In summer its showers are very infrequent, and in a word, Apulia is exposed to the scorching beams of the sun, by virtue both of the dryness of the soil, and of its vicinity to the east; and the inhabitants breathe in an air that feels as if it came from a burning oven. . . . This temperament of the climate is matched by that of the inhabitants; for generally speaking they are of a hot, scorched constitution, with black hair and a brownish or palish skin, meagre, impatient, peevish, watchful, very quick in their way of apprehension, nimble in reasoning and extremely active. They are very subject to ardent fevers, frenzies, pleurisies, madness and other inflammatory diseases. Nay, the heat is so excessive in that country, that I have seen several of the inhabitants urged by it to the last degree of impatience and madness." [16] Baglivi emphasizes in another passage [17] "that there is a greater frequency of melancholic and mad people in Apulia than in any other country of Italy . . . A further confirmation may be taken from the great frequency of mad dogs, whose madness is justly attributed to the scorching heat of the air. But such is the Divine Bounty that those who are bitten by mad dogs are speedily cured by repairing to the Tomb of St. Viti, about 40 miles from Lecce, where the intercession of the Saint procures them a favourable return from the Almighty."

The coast line was colonized by the Greeks and was part of Magna Graecia. Inland the population developed very slowly and remained primitive to this very day; Apulian peasants can still be found living in round huts of the pre-Roman type. The chief city was Taranto, the Greek Taras, the Roman Tarentum. The folk dance that developed in Taranto was the *tarantella* and the spider found in that region the *tarantula*. The disease was attributed to the sting of the spider and was therefore called *tarantismo*. The people suffering from it were *tarantati*, or they were called in a more general way *spezzati*, *schantati*, *minuzzati*, *rotti*, or *tramazzati*.[18] The tarantula occurs all over Italy and in other countries of southern Europe where it is considered a perfectly harmless spider. Baglivi, therefore, points out that the tarantula is venomous in Apulia only and nowhere else.[19]

The disease occurred at the height of the summer heat, in July and August, and particularly during the dog days. People, asleep or awake, would suddenly jump up, feeling an acute pain like the sting of a bee. Some saw the spider, others did not, but they knew that it must be the tarantula. They ran out of the house into the street, to the market place dancing in great excitement. Soon they were joined by others who like them had just been bitten, or by people who had been stung in previous years, for the disease was never quite cured. The poison remained in the body and was reactivated every year by the heat of summer. People were known to have relapsed every summer for thirty years.[20] All ages were affected; a boy of five and a man of ninety-four years had once been bitten, but most tarantati were young people. The disease attacked both sexes, but more women than men. Most patients were "homines rustici similesque femelle," [21] peasant people, but ladies and gentlemen, and even monks and nuns were not spared. All races were attacked. Ferdinandus knew of an Albanian, a gypsy girl and a negro who had been bitten and danced.[22]

Thus groups of patients would gather, dancing wildly in the queerest attire. "Sometimes their fancy leads them to rich clothes, curious vests and necklaces and suchlike ornaments . . . They are most delighted with clothes of a gay color, for the most part red, green, and yellow. On the other hand they cannot endure black; the very sight of it sets them a sighing; and if any of those that stand about them are clad in that color, they are ready to beat them, and bid them be gone." [23] Others would tear their clothes and show their nakedness, losing all sense of modesty. Almost all would hold pieces of red cloth in their hands, waving them, delighted with the sight. "There are some of them that, during the exercise of dancing, are mightily pleased with the green boughs of vines or reeds and wave them about in their hands in the air, or dip them in the water, or bind them about their face and neck." [24] Some called for swords and acted like fencers, others for whips and beat each other. Women called for mirrors, sighed and howled making indecent motions. Some of them had still stranger fancies, liked to be tossed in the air, dug holes in the ground and rolled themselves in the dirt like swine.[25] They all drank wine plentifully and sang and talked like drunken people. And all the while they danced and danced madly to the sound of music.

Music and dancing were the only effective remedies, and people were known to have died within an hour or in a few days because music was not available. A member of Dr. Ferdinandus' own family, his cousin Francesco Franco, died thus within twenty-four hours because no musician could be found after he had been stung. As a rule, however, musicians were at hand. It seems, as a matter of fact, that the spiders were particularly aggressive when the musicians were around, and that music more than the summer heat was responsible for reviving the old poison in the system of former patients. Bands of musicians roamed the country during the summer months with violins, various kinds of pipes, citherns, harps, timbrels, small drums.[26] They played the tarantella, repeating a melody endless times, playing fast. As Baglivi said: [27] "However, this must be taken for a truth, that how much so ever they vary in their particular tunes, yet they all agree in this, to

219

have the notes run over with the greatest quickness imaginable (which quickness of sound is commonly called tarantella)." The musicians stayed in a place for a few days, sometimes for a week, and then went on to the next village. They made good money during the season.

The music was not only instrumental but also vocal, and Kircher has preserved some of the songs. They are love songs, written in Italian dialects, like the following: [28]

> Allu Mari mi portati
> Se voleti che mi sanati.
> Allu Mari, alla via:
> Cosi m'ama la Donna Mia.
> Allu Mari, allu Mari;
> Mentre campo, t'aggio amari.

or like the following: [29]

> Non fù Taranta, nè fù la Tarantella,
> Ma fù lo vino della garratella.
> Dove te mozicò dill'amata dove fù,
> Ohime si fusse gamma, ohime mamma, ohime.

And others sang, repeating the verses endlessly: [30]

> Deu ti mussicau la Tarantella?
> Sotto la Pudia della vanella.

I am quoting these songs in order to illustrate still further what has already become apparent, namely, the sexual character of the disease.

To the tunes of the music the tarantati danced and acted wildly for days on end. It was common for people to go on for four days, sometimes even six days. Ferdinandus even knew of people who had danced for two weeks, and several times a year, but this was unusual.

"They frequently begin to dance about sun rising," to quote Baglivi again,[31] "and some continue in it without intermission till towards eleven in the forenoon. There are, however, some stops made; not from any weariness, but because they observe the mu-

50. TARANTULA. (From Giorgio Baglivi, *Opera omnia*, Nuremberg, 1751.)

Quæ identidem repetunt. Iterum ijs, qui viridi colore afficiuntur.
verbis iucundis, hortos floridos . campos , fyluasque amœnas refpi-
cientibus præcinunt; ijs verò , qui rubris , aut armorum fulgore afficiuntur, modulationes martiales, iambicos, bacchicos, & dithyram-
bos variè diuifos; ijs verò qui aquis gaudent, cantiones amorofas,
flumina, fontes, catarractas refpicientes, atque hifce & fimilibus non
paffio duntaxat Tarantifmo affectorum ; fed & melancholiæ, amo-
ris, iræ, vindictæque affectus mirum eft. quam fedetur.   Verum ne
quicquam in hac arte noftra magnetica curiofarum rerum omififfe
videamur, iftiufmodi antidotariæ Muficæ fpeciem à duobus eximijs
muficis Tarentino & Lupienfi choro præfectis in fuas voces vna
cum faltibus , & fingularum vocum diminutionibus, prout inftru-
mentis concini folent , digeftam , compofitamque hoc loco repræ-
fentare vifum eft.

*Claufulæ Harmonicæ , quas Cytharædi & Aulædi, in cura eorum, qui
Tarantula intoxicati funt, adhibere folent.*

Primus modus Tarentella.

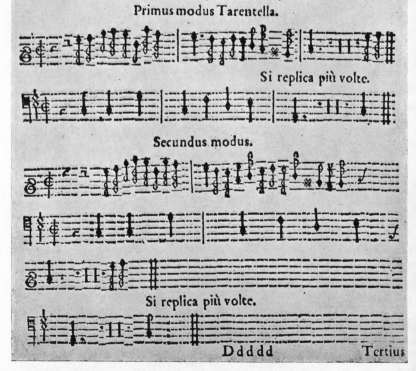

Si replica più volte.

Secundus modus.

Si replica più volte.

51. TARANTELLA. (From Athanasius Kircher, *De arte magnetica*

sical instruments to be out of tune; upon the discovery of which, one would not believe what vehement sighings and anguish at heart they are seized with and in this case they continue till the instrument is got into tune again, and the dance renewed . . . About noon the exercise ceases, and they are covered up in a bed to force out the sweat: When this is done, and the sweat wiped off, they are refreshed with broth, or some such light food; for their extraordinary want of appetite will not allow them to feed higher. About one o'clock after noon, or two at farthest, they renew the exercise as before, and continue it in the manner above mentioned till the evening; then to bed they go again for another sweat: When that is over, and they have got a little refreshment, they lay themselves to sleep."

After having thus danced for a number of days, the people were exhausted—and cured, at least for the time being. But they knew that the poison was in them and that every summer the tunes of the tarantella would revive their frenzy. Many of them, particularly women, did not mind, but liked it. Some were known to have simulated the disease in order to participate in the dances, women in love or those who felt lonely. Many purposely abstained from sexual intercourse in order to have more *deliramenta,* to be more passionate when the time of dancing came.[32] The whole performance was sometimes laughingly called *Il Carnevaletto delle Donne,* the women's little carnival.[33]

The physicians were obviously interested in this strange disease. They accepted the popular theory that attributed it to the sting of the tarantula, but there were difficulties which called for explanation. The spider was venomous in Apulia only. The same tarantula shipped to other parts of the country seemed to lose most of its venom, and what remained acted differently. Baglivi had a rabbit bitten in Naples by an Apulian tarantula. The rabbit died the fifth day but did not dance, although musicians were called and played a great variety of tunes.[34] This was strange because in Apulia a wasp and a rooster had been seen dancing after they had been bitten. And the tarantula herself danced whenever she heard the music.[35] A skeptical physician in Naples had himself bitten in the left arm by two Apulian tarantulae in August 1693 before six witnesses and a public notary. He felt a prick and the arm was somewhat swollen, but otherwise he felt no evil effects.[36] It seemed, therefore, that it was the scorching heat of Apulia that activated the virus and gave it its specific effect. But then, there were other countries just as hot as Apulia where the same tarantula occurred, and yet there was no such thing as tarantism. All this was very mysterious.

Another difficulty that had to be explained was presented by the fact that the poison remained sometimes for decades in the victim's organism without presenting any symptoms except for a short period in the summer. This could be explained, however, in analogy with the syphilis virus. A man could seemingly be cured of syphilis, yet the disease would break out again after many years, which meant that the poison was still in the system. In the case of tarantism the virus was in the body, and what activated it periodically was the heat as well as the music.

The physicians examined a good many patients, but the symptoms they found were very indefinite. Where a bite had actually occurred there was a local wound surrounded by a livid or yellowish circle with some swelling not very different from that caused by other insect bites. Otherwise patients complained about headaches, difficulty of breathing, heart pains, faintings, thirst, lack of appetite, pains in the bones. They frequently said that they felt as if their bones had been broken. Since they all danced, the violent exercise was enough to explain the symptoms.

The physicians also experimented with a variety of treatments. They recommended that the wound be treated like those caused by other venomous animals, by scarifying it with the lancet, or by applying a cupping glass in order to extract the poison. Baglivi suggested cauterization of the wound with a red-hot iron, but never had an opportunity to test it. Internally they gave alexi-pharmaca, antidotes such as treacle or brandy.

The results were not encouraging, and besides the great majority of all patients had no wound. They had been bitten, but in the past. When the tarantati danced at the height of summer, they naturally sweated tremendously, and the physicians thought that this profuse perspiration effected the cure by driving out the poison. And so they made patients sweat without dancing by giving them diaphoretic remedies, but without any result. The doctors, finally, had to admit that music was the only cure, not music at large but the tunes played in Apulia for centuries in the treatment of tarantism. The music, the dances it caused and the resulting perspiration cured the patients, if not permanently, at least temporarily for the season.

As a good iatromechanist, Baglivi had no difficulty in explaining the pathogenesis of the disease and the mechanism of the cure.[37] "This venom," he wrote, "in respect of itself must consist in the highest degree of exaltation; but with respect to the diversity of the constitutions of men, it produces various effects. Among which the principal are condensation and coagulation, and an oppression of the spirits . . . And though the poison of the Tarantula, by activity of its virulent substance does almost dispose the humors to coagulation; yet by virtue of the brisk and lively motion of its constituent parts, it hinders, in some measure, the total coagulation of the humors, and by giving a fillip to the spirits and humors, prevents their final sinking. Nay, sometimes such is the agitation of the spirits, that they degenerate into involuntary and purely spasmodic motions."

On the basis of such a theory it was easy to explain the effect of the music: "It being manifest . . . that music ravishes healthy persons into such actions as imitate the harmony they hear, we easily adjust our opinion of the effects of music in the cure of persons stung by a tarantula. It is probable, that the very swift motion impressed upon the air by musical instruments, and communicated by the air to the skin, and so to the spirits and blood, does, in some measure, dissolve and dispel their growing coagulation; and that the effects of the dissolution increase as the sound itself increases, till, at last, the humors retrieve their primitive fluid state, by virtue of these repeated shakings and vibrations; upon which the patient revives gradually, moves his limbs, gets upon his legs, groans, jumps about with violence, till the sweat breaks and carries off the seeds of the poison."

It seems that tarantism gradually died out during the 18th century. Cases were still reported, particularly after Baglivi's Dissertation had drawn the attention of the entire medical world to the subject. His name carried great weight, and doctors and laymen began to look around wondering whether this strange disease did not occur in their country also. The *Gentlemen's Magazine* published in its September number of 1753 the letter of an Italian music student Stephan Storace who had seen a case in Torre della Annunziata and had played the tarantella for the patient. He wrote the music down and added it to his letter.[38] Other incidental reports came from other countries, but by and large the disease died out. It was found, in addition, that the Apulian tarantula was in no way different from that of other countries and that the symptoms caused by its sting were perfectly harmless. Tarantism was discarded as a myth. Yet it had undoubtedly been a very real disease which for centuries had affected many people. If it was not caused by the venom of a spider, what was its nature?

Ferdinandus gives us a clue.[39] He said that according to some people tarantism was not a disease at all, a view that he refuted immediately with the argument that if tarantism was a mere fiction, there would not be so many poor people, and particularly poor women, spending nearly all their money on the music. They did so because they knew that without the music and the dancing they would be in a very bad condition. Ferdinandus then added that some people considered tarantism *melancholiae seu amentiae quaedam species,* some kind of melancholy or insanity. And this undoubtedly was the correct interpretation. Tarantism was a disease, but it was not caused by the sting of the tarantula. It was a nervous disorder, was a strange neurosis.

But now we must try to explain why people connected this neurosis with the tarantula and why it manifested itself through such queer symptoms. Here again Ferdinandus unwittingly gives us a clue. Discussing the musical treatment of tarantism, he said that its origin was unknown, but then he added that the Greek traditions had always been very strong in Apulia. It once had been a part of Magna Graecia and in this very region the two great Greeks Pythagoras and Archytas had been teaching.[40]

Without being aware of it Ferdinandus put his finger on the right spot. We have seen the great part played by music in the School of Pythagoras. In the same region ancient deities such as Dionysos, Cybele, Demeter and others were worshiped, and in many of these cults—particularly that of Dionysos—orgiastic rites of a decidedly erotic character were performed. People danced madly to the sound of music, dressed in bright clothes with garlands of vine leaves, waving the thyrsus, uttering obscene words, tearing their clothes, whipping each other, drinking wine. The analogy between these rites and the symptoms of tarantism is striking. What is the connection?

Christianity came late to Apulia and found a primitive and conservative population in which ancient beliefs and customs were deeply rooted. In competition with paganism Christianity had to adjust itself in many ways in order to win over the population. Ancient holidays were preserved and made to commemorate Christian events. Churches were erected on ancient sites of worship among the ruins of temples. Saints took over functions and attributes of pagan deities. Elements of ancient cults such as processions were taken over in Christianized form. There were limits, however, that the Church could not well overstep. It could not assimilate the orgiastic rites of the cult of Dionysos but had to fight them. And yet these very rites that appealed to the most elementary instincts were the most deeply rooted. They persisted, and we can well imagine that people gathered secretly to perform the old dances and all that went with them. In doing so they sinned, until one day—we do not know when but it must have been during the Middle Ages—the meaning of the dances had changed. The old rites appeared as symptoms of a disease. The music, the dances, all that wild orgiastic behavior were legitimized. The people who indulged in these exercises were no longer sinners but the poor victims of the tarantula.

According to all medical testimonies, Apulia with its inbred population had a high incidence of mental diseases, and there can be no doubt that the great majority of all tarantati were neurotics. Tarantism was a neurosis peculiar to that region. It is at the same time one more example of the survival of pagan institutions in the Christian world and a particularly interesting one on account of its medical and musical implications.

NOTES

1. I Samuel, 17, 23.
2. See L. Edelstein, Greek Medicine in its Relation to Religion and Magic, *Bulletin of the Institute of the History of Medicine,* 1937, vol. V, p. 234 ff. where the following passages have been collected.
3. De morbis acutis et chronicis, ed. I. C. Amman, 1709, p. 555.
4. Loeb Classical Library, 1927, vol. I, pp. 352–354, translation by J. C. Rolfe.
5. Caelius Aurelianus, *l.c.*
6. Liber Usualis Missae et Officii, Festa Junii 24.

7. In order that thy servants may sing with relaxed fibers the marvels of thy deeds, absolve, oh St. John, the guilt of the polluted lip.

8. Johannes Wolf, Bonaiutus de Casentino, ein Dichter-Komponist um 1300, *Acta Musicologica*, 1937, vol. IX, fasc. I–II, pp. 1–5. I am indebted to Mr. L. Ellinwood of the Music Department of Michigan State College for drawing my attention to this piece.

9. May the bowels thus be washed and the cesspool of the mind purge itself of every evil. Care of the skin is worthy when it brings the gift of health to both aspects of man. When the sensitive and intellectual faculties are preserved there is good hope for consolation.

10. Blood taken and redeemed may keep us joyful. May the eternal glory of the heavens thereby be wished for and granted.

11. First published in a collection entitled *Frottole libro tertio,* a copy of which is preserved in the Biblioteca Marucelliana in Florence. See Emil Vogel, *Bibliothek der gedruckten weltlichen Vocalmusik Italiens, Aus den Jahren 1500–1700,* 1892, vol. II, p. 374 ff. The text of the Frottola was reprinted by L. Joseph, *Schweizerische Medizinische Wochenschrift,* 1937, p. 1004.

12. What violence and rage of so great a disease, what plague, what force harasses the mind, what evil creeps, sweet poison devours the marrow.

13. Epiphanius Ferdinandus, *Centum Historiae seu Observationes et Casus Medici,* Venetiis, 1621. Historia LXXXI, seu casus octuagesimus primus, De morsu Tarantulae, pp. 248–268.

14. Dissertatio de Anatome, Morsu, et Effectibus Tarantulae, reprinted in the various editions of the *Opera Omnia Medico-practica et Anatomica.* An English translation, A Dissertation of the Anatomy, Bitings and other Effects of the venemous Spider, call'd Tarantula was published with *The Practice of Physick.* The passages quoted in the following are from the 2nd English edition, London 1723.

15. The edition I have been using is the *Editio secunda post Romanam multo correctior,* Coloniae Agrippinae, 1643.

16. *L.c.,* p. 317.

17. *L.c.,* p. 365.

18. Ferdinandus, *l.c.,* p. 258.

19. *L.c.,* p. 335.

20. Ferdinandus, *l.c.,* p. 258.

21. *L.c.,* p. 264.

22. *L.c.,* pp. 261–262.

23. Baglivi, *l.c.,* p. 347.

24. Baglivi, *l.c.,* p. 346.

25. Baglivi, *l.c.,* pp. 331, 346.

26. The instruments are described in Kircher's book, *l.c.,* p. 765.

27. *L.c.,* p. 348.

28. Carry me to the sea if you wish to cure me. To the sea, to the sea, thus my be-

loved loves me. To the sea, to the sea, as long as I live I shall love thee. Kircher, *l.c.*, p. 763.

29. It was neither a big nor a small tarantula; it was the wine from the flask. Where did it bite you, tell me, beloved, where it was. Oh, if it was your leg, oh mamma! Kircher, *l.c.*, p. 760.

30. Where did the tarantula bite you? Under the fringe of the skirt. Kircher, *ibidem.*

31. *L.c.*, p. 344.

32. Ferdinandus, *l.c.*, p. 260.

33. Baglivi, *l.c.*, p. 335.

34. *L.c.*, p. 350.

35. Ferdinandus, *l.c.*, p. 261.

36. Baglivi, *l.c.*, p. 361.

37. See *l.c.*, pp. 366–373.

38. A German translation of the letter was published in *Hamburgisches Magazin, oder gesammelte Schriften, Aus der Naturforschung und den angenehmen Wissenschaften überhaupt,* Des dreyzehnten Bandes erstes Stück, pp. 3–8, Hamburg and Leipzig, 1754.

39. *L.c.*, p. 254.

40. *L.c.*, p. 266: cum enim nos semper grecissemus, nam haec nostra Regio dicebatur Magna Graecia, in qua olim Pythagoras et Archytas, praestantissimi Graecorum, summa ac admirabili auditorum frequentia docuerunt.

CHAPTER XII

Civilization Against Disease

MAN HAS at all times been ravaged by disease. Parasites have assailed him; the physical and chemical forces of his environment have constantly interfered with the normal course of his life. When his organism grew old, his resistance to these hostile forces lessened and in the end he succumbed to them. But at all times he reacted against them. Nature had endowed him, like other animals, with the most powerful urge, the drive to preserve his life and to perpetuate his kind.

Like other animals also, man at first reacted against disease instinctively, rubbing an aching limb, scratching an itching sore, moving close to the fire to relieve a pain in the back. Instinctively he sought foods that made him strong and herbs that cured him when he felt sick. Instinctively he evaded dangers that threatened him.

But nature endowed man with more than instincts. It gave him a better brain than other animals, the power to observe and to reason about things, to remember them and to communicate his experience to others by means of language. Great discoveries must have been made at a very early date. For thousands of years people broke their legs while hunting in the forest. When such an accident occurred, the victim crawled back to his cave or hut or was carried by his companions. Weeks passed by, the fracture healed but the leg was shorter and the man a cripple, unable to hunt, dependent on his fellow men. And then one day somebody had the idea of stretching the broken leg so as to prevent it from becoming shorter. Painful as the procedure was to the victim, he pulled the broken end, and he soon noticed that the leg contracted again as soon as it was released. Then he took a piece of bark or a strip of wood, made a splint, attached it to the broken leg, and thus forced it to remain extended. As a result the victim recovered without being crippled. This was one of the greatest surgical discoveries that could ever be made. It must have occurred not once but several times, spontaneously, in various parts of the world, as a result of man's powers of observation and his inventiveness.

Civilization gradually developed. Man gained power over nature, learned to direct its forces in order to make his life safer. He tilled the soil, bred animals, cut his way through the jungle and irrigated the desert. Medicine, the art of preserving and restoring health, is one aspect of human civilization. Like agriculture, it is an endeavor to preserve life and make it more secure. Its history reflects the general history of civilization, as we have seen on every page of this book. As civilization advanced, man became able to fight disease more and more effectively, and in this struggle medicine was his chief weapon.

Medicine—I am using the term in its broadest sense—always had two elements. From the beginning it was a craft, practised by craftsmen who worked with their hands and who had to be skillful in order to do a good job. Manual procedures were often transmitted independently from literature through practical instruction, from father to son, from master to pupil. Surgeons always travelled more than other medical men, in the wake of armies; and in foreign lands they saw new operative techniques, learned them from their colleagues, brought them home and taught them to their own disciples. Thus it is often difficult to trace the history of a surgical operation. The knowledge of it seems to jump from one country to another, and we may not be able to find any literary link.

Craftsmanship was by no means limited to surgery. The ancient physician gathered the herbs and minerals he needed for drugs, prepared his own composite remedies, made salves, pills, electuaria, syrups. He performed fumigations and irrigations on the patient, examined him not only with his eyes but with his hands, feeling the pulse, the tension of the skin, searching for tumors. And later he learned to handle more and more complicated diagnostic instruments and apparatuses.

The craft of medicine was certainly not independent from its theory, but it nevertheless represents to a certain extent a separate line of development, its empirical line. Many surgical operations such as the suture of wounds, reduction of dislocated joints, splinting of fractured bones, trephining of the skull, were performed for thousands of years with hardly any modification. They were devised empirically, at a time when anatomical knowledge was scanty. But they worked; they served their purpose and were applied irrespective of theories. In a similar way, many drugs were given for thousands of years on the basis of experience. Once the purgative effect of castor-oil, rhubarb, or coloquinths and the narcotic effect of opium had been observed, they were used successfully no matter what the pharmacological theory of the time was. The theory had to adapt itself to the facts. Diets devised by Hippocratic physicians for the sick are still used today in basically the same composition. The Greeks knew that they helped; we know why they help, and throughout the centuries patients were benefited by them.

There was always a relation between the craft of medicine and the technology of the time. Operations can be performed with bronze knives, but steel knives were much better. A skull can be opened with a cylindrical saw operated by hand, but an electrical trephine works faster and is more precise. A cautery can be heated on coal, but an electrical cautery can be maintained accurately at a uniform temperature. Medical techniques were always greatly improved in periods when people were mechanically minded. It is not by accident that the obstetrical forceps was invented in the 17th century.

But medicine is not only a craft; it is also part of the general learning of a period and reflects its general outlook on life, its *Weltanschauung*. Disease appeared as a process of nature which had to be studied like other natural phenomena. Primitive people already knew that they could fight disease much more effectively if they not only followed traditional routines but were cognizant of etiology and pathogenesis, that is, of the causes and mechanism of the disease. Once the causes were known, individuals could protect themselves. If the disease had broken out, the treatment could be directed at removing the cause, for *causa remota cessat effectus*. Once the pathogenesis of a disease was known, it became possible to direct the treatment and the healing power of the organism in the right direction.

Disease was interpreted with the aid of all intellectual resources available at the time, and in previous chapters we have discussed the long way that medicine had to go from magic to religion, philosophy, and finally to science. Medicine fully participated in the great rise of natural science, and by doing so became infinitely more effective than in the past. In the new medical science civilization had forged a weapon that could be used in an attempt to liberate man from the age-old bond of disease.

Civilization is a very complex phenomenon. It has both material and spiritual aspects. A nation may produce great painters, poets and philosophers but cannot be considered truly civilized as long as its infants die like flies and the mass of the people live in misery and starvation. Nobody, on the other hand, would consider a society civilized merely because it had attained a high standard of living and good health conditions. Civilization requires the cultivation of all those spiritual values that make life truly humane and thus worth living. The part that medicine can play is limited, yet medicine is important because it greatly contributes to human welfare and helps to create conditions for the development of culture.

Like civilization at large, medicine is very young. Five thousand years is a very short period in the perspectives of history, but nevertheless a great deal was achieved and health conditions improved considerably, at least in the Western world. Still more encouraging is the fact that progress now comes much more rapidly than in the past. More advances were made in the last hundred years than in the four thousand nine hundred that preceded them. We may therefore expect further impressive gains in the near future, and disease may well be eradicated a few centuries from now.

It would be a great mistake, however, to give all the credit for improved health conditions to medical science. Other factors have played an equally important part. The dreaded leprosy practically disappeared from Western Europe because the Black Death wiped most lepers out. Plague itself disappeared from Europe in the early 18th century for reasons that are not quite apparent. Sanitary measures such as widespread quarantine were undoubtedly helpful, but the general sanitary condition of cities was still extremely bad; they were all infested with rats.

The general death-rate dropped steadily from the 17th century on, at a time when medical science was still undeveloped. This is particularly striking in the case of a rapidly growing city like London for which very impressive figures are available, some of which have already been quoted in a previous chapter: [1]

CIVILIZATION AND DISEASE

Years	Population	Annual deaths per 1,000 population
1681–1690	530,000	42
1746–1755	653,000	35
1846–1855	2,362,236	25

Sanitation alone could not explain these figures. The improved conditions must to a large extent be the result of a rising standard of living. While industrialization created new health hazards and for a long time was responsible for atrocious working and living conditions, it ultimately raised the living standards of millions of people, and today health conditions in many countries are far better among the industrial than among the rural population.

Civilization fights disease in many ways, but medicine nevertheless is its most powerful weapon. Smallpox, once one of the great killers that wiped out entire populations, declined in the 18th century, when the method of inoculation was introduced, and became a totally preventable disease with Jenner's discovery of vaccination. The methods of immunization worked out for rabies, diphtheria, tetanus, typhoid fever, cholera, yellow fever, and a number of other diseases have greatly reduced their incidence and will ultimately overcome them entirely. Tuberculosis has lost much of its terror and will die out in a not too distant future, at least in the economically advanced countries. The venereal diseases are receding rapidly also because we know their etiology and pathogenesis and have developed effective treatments. These two diseases are being overcome rapidly wherever the population is sufficiently advanced socially to accept stringent legislation. Pneumonia, only yesterday a major cause of death, is curable today by chemotherapy. Puerperal fever and other deadly streptococcus infections will soon be considered diseases of the past.

Great advances were made not only in the field of infectious diseases. The insulin treatment of diabetes and the liver treatment of pernicious anemia has kept alive thousands of people who, infallibly, would have died only a short while ago. The discovery of vitamins has made it possible to cure and prevent such diseases as rickets, scurvy, pellagra and beriberi. Diseases of the endocrine system were brought under control when the nature and function of the hormones became known. Surgery greatly improved its operative results and succeeded in standardizing its methods in such a way that major operations can be performed safely by every qualified surgeon. The improved methods of blood transfusion save many human lives and are particularly important in a mechanical age when accidents have become a major cause of death.

The general health conditions of a nation can be measured and expressed in figures. The general death-rate indicates the number of people dying in a year for every 1,000 population. It has been decreasing steadily. In most countries it was hardly ever under 50 in the 18th century, while today it is between 8 and 15 in the countries of Western civilization. It was 17.6 in the United States in 1900 and was reduced to 11.5 in 1936. These latter figures tell us that in 1936 not less than 750,000 human lives were saved in the United States that would have been lost in 1900. This certainly is an impressive number.

In the past, mortality was particularly high among infants, and the improvements made in this field are most spectacular. The infantile death-rate, that is the number of children dying in the first year of life for every 1,000 children born, is today between 30 and 70 in most civilized countries. It was ten times higher in the 18th century.

As a result of improved health conditions and particularly as a result of the reduced infantile mortality, the average life expectancy has increased considerably. A child born in Europe in the

15th century had an average life expectancy of from twenty to twenty-five years, while it is between sixty and sixty-six today in the economically advanced countries.

There is no doubt that civilization has succeeded in making life infinitely less hazardous than it was in the past, but the task is by no means completed. We mentioned before that improvements have been achieved only in a relatively small number of countries and that over one half of the population of the world still lives under atrocious health conditions and has not benefited by the progress of medical science. Their problem is particularly difficult because health cannot be brought to them from outside while they are kept on a low standard of living. To immunize colonial people against disease with one hand and exploit them into starvation with the other is a grim joke. Economic freedom and education are the foundations of every kind of public health work. Without them all efforts remain futile.

Medical science is still facing a large number of unsolved problems. Even in the field of infectious and contagious diseases where the greatest advances have been made so far, there are still many questions for which we have no answer. The influenza pandemic of 1918–1919 took a death toll of ten million lives, and since influenza invades the world with great regularity once in a generation, we may expect another devastating pandemic at any time. And we are hardly better prepared for it than we were in 1918. Poliomyelitis has increased in recent years, and we can do very little to prevent young people from being crippled by it. The common cold and its complications do not kill people, but they create more temporary disability than any other disease, and we are still unable to prevent or cure them.

Since more people become old today than in the past, more people die from the diseases of maturity and old age. We have already seen that cancer is the second cause of death in the United States;

diseases of heart and circulation take first rank and the mortality from them is very high. Not content with just killing their victims, these two groups of diseases handicap and disable them for long periods of time, as do also arthritis, rheumatism and a number of other chronic diseases.

Such chronic ailments have sometimes been called "wear-and-tear diseases." They develop when the individual is getting older and their course is accelerated by the stress and strain of modern life. The machine simply breaks down. We may not be able to prevent them entirely, but we may learn how to postpone them. We can already prolong the life of such patients quite considerably.

Thus medical science still has many great problems to solve, but research is carried on vigorously in laboratories and at the bedside of patients. Our medical schools are no longer mere teaching institutions but active centers of research. While the young student is trained to be a physician, he is brought into close contact with medical scientists who are engaged in research. He becomes a scientist himself. Independent research institutions like the Rockefeller Institute for Medical Research in New York and Princeton were established in the course of our century in a number of countries. They are supported either by public funds or by private endowments. Modern scientific research is costly, but governments should realize that money spent on medical research is a self-liquidating investment that brings high dividends. Every medical advance achieved reduces the incidence of illness and by preserving human lives saves society considerable financial outlay. It is a truism to state that the prevention of illness is infinitely cheaper than its cure, but it cannot be repeated often enough because hardly any government acts according to this simple rule.

Health conditions have greatly improved in the economically advanced countries and this is very gratifying, but we should never be satisfied with the results achieved. We should always keep the failures and short-comings in mind. We should not rejoice about the fact that we had fewer cases of tuberculosis last year than we had the year before, but should feel concerned that we still have so many cases. We must not think only in terms of rates but also in absolute figures. We may have a low infantile mortality rate in the United States, but we still lose many thousands of children needlessly, and this is most disturbing. We may have a relatively low maternal death-rate, but nevertheless thousands of American families are deprived every year of the wife and mother without necessity. If we stop thinking merely in rates and try to visualize for a moment the anguish and sorrow created in so many families by these maternal deaths, we realize that we have no cause for rejoicing where there is still so much to be done.

We must never say that health conditions are good, but must rather ask ourselves constantly whether they are as good as they could be. The answer is decidedly: no. We are confronted by great gaps in our knowledge of disease and are still without methods of effective treatment against many of them. Where this is the case we cannot expect great results and must concentrate our efforts on research. But already we know a great deal. We know the cause and pathogenesis of many diseases and have effective treatments against them. Yet they are still among us. Every society still carries an enormous burden of unnecessary illness, and in the United States it has been estimated that one-third of all deaths are premature, that the individuals could have lived much longer if they had had all the benefits of medical science. We could eliminate venereal diseases in a couple of years at the cost of one or two battleships, but we are not doing so. There is no excuse for still having cases of smallpox and diphtheria; an epidemic of typhoid or dysentery is no longer a catastrophe but a scandal.

We must also keep the minor ailments in mind: those that do not kill but disable. In the United States the average worker loses approximately 8 days a year as a result of illness. This is much less than in the past. In 1873 Pettenkofer estimated that the average inhabitant of Munich lost 20 days a year as a result of illness.[2] Yet these 8 days still mean that American industry is deprived every year of 400,000,000 man-days.[3]

The war of 1914–1918 drew the attention of the people to the fact that in spite of progress health conditions were by no means satisfactory. In the present war the draft examinations have revealed that almost one-half of the young people examined could not meet strict health requirements. Their defects were in many cases of a minor nature and could be remedied easily, but the very fact that they existed and had not been attended to by the individuals is a sad comment on conditions in a country that possesses almost all the personnel and equipment that are needed.

Medical science has progressed and health conditions have improved, but by no means in the same proportion. Medical science has infinitely more to give than the people actually receive. The causes of this maladjustment are easily apparent and have been discussed so many times that here I will summarize the argument very briefly.

Health conditions are determined by a variety of factors. One, and a very important one, is social and economic. Poverty is the curse of mankind. In a world that could produce all the food that the people could possibly consume; at a time when science is advanced enough to exploit the resources of nature systematically and to produce all the commodities that could be used—the great majority of all inhabitants of the earth are still on a level that does not permit them to lead healthy lives.

Poverty remains the chief cause of disease, and it is a factor which is beyond the immediate control of medicine. The remedy is obvious. The standard of living must be raised, not only in a few countries of the West, but in India, China, Africa, all over the world. Nations cannot prosper at the expense of other nations, groups at the expense of other groups. The world has become so small that misery in one nation is bound to affect the others. Standards can be raised if we at last learn to apply principles of science to the basic processes of social life, to production, distribution and consumption, if we plan social life along scientific lines and on a world-wide scale.

Health conditions are also determined by educational standards. Ignorance too is a major cause of disease. Health cannot be brought to the people from outside; it cannot be forced on them. When the Russians reorganized their medical services after the Revolution, they did so under the slogan: "The people's health is the concern of the people themselves," and their entire health work is carried out with broad participation of the population. Unless the people are able and willing to accept their physicians' advice and to cooperate with them, our efforts must fail. Education, however, consists of more than knowledge of reading and writing and a few half-baked notions about disease. It must impart a positive attitude toward health, the acceptance of individual responsibility toward society, and must overcome customs and prejudices which, sanctioned by tradition, nevertheless seriously interfere with a healthy life. It is a difficult task, one that requires much psychological understanding and tact, but education—general as well as health education—is the foundation of all health work.

Health conditions, finally are determined by the effectiveness of medical services. Medical science is wasted unless it can be applied without reservation. We need a system of health services that reaches everybody, healthy and sick, rich and poor, and there is no reason why we should not be able to establish such a system. Greater organizational problems have been solved and are being solved, particularly in these very days of war.

What we need is the iron determination to be a sound and healthy nation, free from the bonds of disease, as far as this is pos-

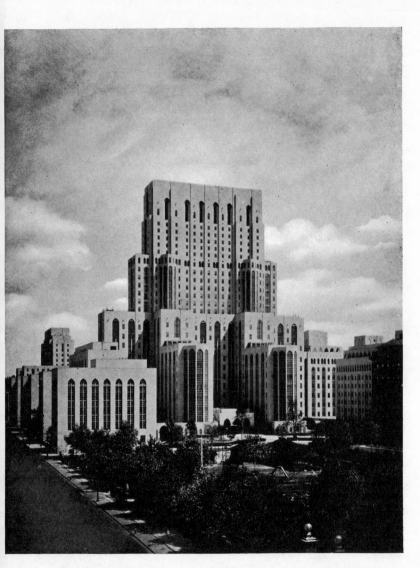

52. A MODERN MEDICAL CENTER. New York Hospital and Cornell Medical College. (Photo by Sigurd Fischer.)

sible. We must also be aware of the fact that conditions have greatly changed in the last hundred years. After two industrial revolutions the structure of society is different from what it was in the past. Medicine has also greatly changed, as a result of its progress. It has become highly technical and calls for the cooperative efforts of general practitioners and specialists, for the wide use of clinics and hospitals. A new medicine serving a new society requires new forms of service. We must break down the artificial barriers between preventive and curative medicine. It is wasteful to erect highly efficient health centers that reach and advise the people and then, at the crucial moment when patients are in need of some treatment, be forced to dismiss them with the words: go and see your doctor—the doctor that so many of them do not have.

The task of medicine is to promote health, to prevent disease, to treat the sick when prevention has broken down and to rehabilitate the people after they have been cured. These are highly social functions and we must look at medicine as basically a social science. Medicine is merely one link in a chain of social welfare institutions that every civilized country must develop. If we have a maladjustment today, it is to a large extent due to the fact that we have neglected the sociology of medicine. For a long time we concentrated our efforts on scientific research and assumed that the application of its results would take care of itself. It did not, and the technology of medicine has outrun its sociology.

This is not the place to discuss the reorganization of medical services,[4] but in the civilized society of tomorrow every family will have not only its family doctor but also its family health center from which it will be entitled to receive all the advice and help it may need as a public service, and with which it will cooperate in upholding the health of the nation. The physician will become a public servant—scientist, social worker and educator—and medicine will increasingly shift the emphasis from disease to health.

The problem of financing such health services is secondary.

Much more difficult economic problems have been solved. We have all the money we need when we are attacked by a ruthless enemy. Disease is also an enemy. Its attack may be less spectacular but is just as pernicious as any that occurs in actual warfare, and we certainly can find the comparatively small funds required to fight this war to a victorious end. The health and welfare of every individual is the concern of society, and human solidarity beyond the boundaries of nationality, race, and creed is a true criterion of civilization.

NOTES

1. See Pettenkofer, *The Value of Health to a City,* Baltimore, 1941, p. 30.
2. *L.c.,* p. 21 ff.
3. The figures are from a memorandum of Medical Administration Service in New York, by Kingsley Roberts and Martin W. Brown, issued in 1941.
4. I have done it in a number of publications such as *Medicine and Human Welfare,* Yale University Press, New Haven, 1941.

Epilogue

IT SEEMS futile to write about civilization at the very moment when it appears to be collapsing, when a war is raging that embraces the globe, and when all the resources of intelligence, of human skill, and natural wealth seem to be mobilized for destruction. And yet we must always remember that civilization is a very young phenomenon in the history of mankind, and that reversals into primitive savagery are bound to occur. Much has been achieved in the short period of five thousand years. Cultural values have been created that no bomb can destroy. There is more freedom, more justice, more health in the world than in the past— yet still not enough, and that is why there is a war.

What happened in the limited field of medicine seems to have happened in the world at large: technology outran sociology. We have created ingenious machines but not the social and economic organization that an industrial society requires. We have built means of transportation that overbridge the continents, but not the apparatus that ensures peaceful cooperation between nations. While we reduced the size of the world, we also confined our thinking in terms of narrow and selfish nationalism. The machine age calls for social and economic adjustments not just in the medical field but everywhere.

Terrible as this war is, its very destructiveness shows symptoms that appear as the birthpains of a new world. It is a revolutionary war. Oppressed nations and oppressed groups are or will be fighting for political and economic independence, for freedom and justice, for the right to work and through their labor to acquire the security that was denied them in the past.

We do not know how long this war will last, whether it will be the final or only one more episode in the conflict that became acute in the beginning of our century. We are impatient because our span of life is so short and we would like to see the outcome. But history beats in longer periods than a man's heart.

The more I study history, the more faith I have in the future of mankind, and the less doubt as to the ultimate result of the present conflict. The step will be taken from the competitive to the cooperative society, democratically ruled on scientific principles, to a society in which all will have equal duties and equal rights, not only on paper but in fact. We may not see it, but our children or their children will. While we are struggling, the foundations are being laid for a new and better civilization.

Index

PHOENIX BOOKS
in Science

PHOENIX SCIENCE SERIES

PHOENIX BOOKS
in History